EFFECTIVE COMMUNICATION IN HEALTH CARE

A Supervisor's Handbook

Harry E. Munn, Jr.
and
Norman Metzger

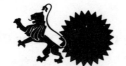

AN ASPEN PUBLICATION
Rockville, Maryland
London
1981

Library of Congress Cataloging in Publication Data

Munn, Harry E.
Effective communication in health care.

Includes bibliographies and index.
1. Health facilities—Personnel management.
2. Communication in personnel management.
3. Supervision of employees. I. Metzger, Norman,
1924-   . II. Title [DNLM: 1. Personnel administration,
Hospital. 2. Communication. WX 159 M966c]
RA971.35.M86   362.1'068'3   81-1387
ISBN: 0-89443-356-3.   AACR2

Copyright © 1981 by Aspen Systems Corporation

Library of Congress Catalog Card Number: 81-1387
ISBN: 0-89443-356-3

Printed in the United States of America

2 3 4 5

To my mother, who has also been my friend; and to Scott, my son, who has given me more support than he will ever know.
Harry E. Munn, Jr.

To my family, a source of continuing support and love.
Norman Metzger

Table of Contents

Preface

Communication is as necessary to an organization as the bloodstream is to a person. Just as the bloodstream must flow unhindered, communication must flow freely. The bloodstream must be responsive to the internal needs of the body. Similarly, communication must be responsive to the internal needs of the organization. This communicative responsiveness requires one to develop an ability to communicate clearly, concisely, and with understanding.

Based on these precepts, this hospital supervisor's handbook is intended for use in hospitals at all levels of supervision. It is meant to be practical and concise. It was written for the following reasons:

1. Supervisors are constantly exchanging information via communication, but they may have only limited knowledge of interpersonal or small group communication processes.
2. The communicative behavior of supervisors with and among other health care professionals and patients will ultimately affect the mental and physical well-being of their patients.
3. Supervisors can improve their communicative knowledge and behavior only through instruction in interpersonal and small group processes.
4. Supervisors have a professional need to be able to diagnose communicative illness and then be able to employ appropriate treatment.
5. Supervisors must be able to apply this treatment, if necessary, in a health care setting.
6. Supervisors might have an abundant supply of medical and technical knowledge, but communication is the only tool they

have with which to exchange this knowledge with others. To be able to share and understand information is the only way an individual or organization can maintain excellent communicative health.

Harry E. Munn, Jr.
and
Norman Metzger
April 1981

Acknowledgments

Grateful acknowledgment is extended to the following friends, from North Carolina State University, who have offered me ideas and suggestions for preparing this book: Chuck Amato, Milton Bliss, Donna J. Dampier, Ann Harris, Betty Knott, Becky Leonard, Nancy Robbins McGranahan, Bo Rein, John Stone, and Charlotte Swart; and to Susan Whisnant of Fairmont Foods.

Further appreciation goes to three special friends: Dr. Bill Conboy of the University of Kansas, who, early in my career, provided me with a solid foundation for understanding organizational communication; Dr. Bill Franklin of North Carolina State University, who inspired me to dream and share personal experiences in the course of writing this book; and Deborah Briley of Cary, North Carolina, who, over the past two years, provided me with encouragement, understanding, and support.

Harry E. Munn, Jr.

A special acknowledgment is overdue, after my first six books, to the many interested and interesting students who have peopled my classes over the past 25 years and who have taught me how to communicate.

Norman Metzger

Chapter 1

How to Communicate for Change

CHAPTER OBJECTIVES

The purpose of this chapter is to enable you to CHANGE your communicative behavior in a *positive* direction. After studying the material you should be able to:

Confer more closely with coworkers and employees.

Have an understanding of the role of the supervisor as an agent of change.

Anticipate and understand why employees may resist change.

Notice and respond to the feedback of coworkers and employees.

Gain insights into the psychological principles of communication.

Examine ways of overcoming resistance to needed change.

INTRODUCTION

If there is a single consistency in today's complex health care industry, it is the move toward change. Supervisors must initiate changes at a faster rate than ever before. These changes will touch the organizational structure, personnel policies, procedures, equipment, techniques, technologies, and, in general, the way health care is delivered. The supervisor has a key role in the communications grid. No matter what the change may be, the average employee will be suspicious and often resistant. To the employee in a department, there is no such thing as an insignificant change. Change implies a move from the old, comfortable, and mastered way to an unknown and threatening way. The best way to introduce the subject of communicating for change is to explore the normal reaction to the announcement of change: resistance.

RESISTANCE TO CHANGE

Resistance is behavior intended to protect the employee or group of employees from the effects of real or imagined change. Resistance is protective and often defensive in nature; it arises from either a real or an imagined threat to the security of the individual or group. It is associated with feelings that range from hostility and aggression to apathy and withdrawal. Not fully understanding how the change will affect them, employees feel suspicious and threatened. There are numerous conditions under which employees tend to resist change:

- When the nature of the change and its effects are not clearly communicated and understood by those affected. Yet, the communication of full information is not in and of itself a guarantee of the elimination of resistance.

- When employees are not prepared for the change. It is disastrous for an institution to announce a critical change to employees who have not been forewarned.

- When employees have not been consulted in advance regarding the necessity for change and have not been included in discussions of alternatives to unproductive procedures or methods.

- When information is distorted, especially if employees have felt uncomfortable and threatened in past work situations. Employees have long memories. Present assurances do not easily eradicate past disappointments.

- When the change is made on personal grounds, rather than because of impersonal requirements of the group or the institution.

- When the change ignores established norms or customs of the group.

- When excessive work pressure is involved in the change. Employees are ever alert to the possibility that change will result in additional work, unfair distribution of the workload, or speedup.

- When the planning of change fails to consider in detail exactly how the change will be brought about. Poor planning will ensure a disaster.

- When insufficient consideration is given to problems that are likely to arise and to the ways to deal with them.

- When there is fear of failure or when the change is seen as inadequate or ineptly managed.

- When it is not obvious what was wrong with the old way of doing things and why the change is needed.

Once people do things in a certain way, they form habits. Change requires a gradual weaning away from the old habits and an alteration of attitudes. Attitudes, for the most part, can be changed only by experience—not as the result of facts. Almost every attempt to introduce change sets up a countervailing force familiarly called "resistance to change," which is initiated by the employee whose job security, habits, or relationships seem to be threatened. Such resistance takes the form of anxious queries, wild rumors of impending disaster, grievances, noncooperation, slowdowns, refusal to meet new goals, or subtle group behavior to discredit the new system.[1]

One observer has questioned the concept of resistance to change and sees it more as resentment or anxiety over the way change is introduced. Trying to convince someone of the advantages of the new method often sounds like criticism of the old, which the employee likes because it is familiar or even because that employee sponsored it originally. More than one supervisor has flatly rejected a change, saying either in anger or in hurt that there is nothing wrong with the performance of the department. Sometimes a change is introduced in a way that appears to threaten established work habits and relationships; it thus never gets a chance to be accepted in its own right. Many supervisors have made a new process turn out to be just as impractical as they predicted it would be.[2]

OVERCOMING RESISTANCE TO CHANGE

Recent studies indicate that supervisors can best initiate change when they:

- use resistance as a diagnostic symptom to get at its cause;
- use feedback, the release of feelings, and the blowing off of steam to air resistance, to bring it out in the open;
- allow the groups involved to make some decisions, within defined limits, on how to implement the change and on how problems will be handled;
- build a trusting work climate, that is, get and give honest answers to questions that relate to policy and procedures;
- communicate, discuss, encourage feedback, and help people gather facts pointing to the need for change as related to their own problems and needs;
- use group norms and customs in planning and implementing change;
- use two-way communication to help those affected develop (1) their own understanding of the need for change, (2) an explicit awareness of how they feel about the change, and (3) an understanding of what can be done about their feelings.[3]

The supervisor's role in overcoming resistance to change starts with the key questions: What is my plan for communicating change? What is my plan for ameliorating the effect of the change on the personnel involved?

It is essential that the reasons for the change be communicated in detail. Do not mask or rationalize these reasons. If change is introduced to reduce costs or increase productivity, state it out front. The employees must understand the impact on their own individual jobs. Essential to the selling of change is the encouragement of an exchange of concerns and information, including the setting up of conditions under which employees are assured their questions will be answered.

A simple plan is to hold a group meeting where the reasons for and the details of the change are explained. This can be followed up with smaller group meetings. In these smaller meetings, the immediate supervisor will explore problems and concerns with subordinates and attempt to ameliorate any apprehension. This can be followed with written communications to all employees. Of course, the supervisors must be trained in advance of the change.

THE SUPERVISOR AS A CHANGE AGENT

Good communication is essential to good employee relations. The supervisor who does not communicate properly will often have an unproductive group. Reliable information is at the heart of communication. If supervisors are not *in* on things, how can they be effective communicators? It is essential that supervisors know what is going on within the institution, what others expect of them, and what is planned for the future.

A willingness to include supervisors in the planning stage is one hallmark of an effective organization. If supervisors know what is expected and why, they can be more productive communicators. They must give meaning to policy and procedure changes in the day-to-day work arena. Employees are quick to understand when supervisors merely mouth institutional policy rather than back it.

A downward flow of formal communications is typical of most institutions. Too often, certain levels of the management hierarchy are bypassed, leading to problems. Supervisors who are bypassed may feel that they are unnecessary links in the chain and fall into negative patterns of working against the organization. Supervisors cannot support what they do not understand or have not been consulted about.

Let us step back at this point and substitute for the term *supervisor* the word *employee*. It is easy to see how the employee's lack of understanding and participation will result in counterproductive behavior.

PSYCHOLOGICAL PRINCIPLES OF COMMUNICATION

There are certain psychological principles of communication that operate in the supervisor-subordinate relationship:

- Whenever two people or groups of people come together, communication goes on. It is patently clear that no one can prevent people from communicating when they are in contact with each other. It is only the direction, quantity, and effectiveness of communication that can be controlled.

- In all communication, listening is as important as talking. Communication is a complete and closed circle. Listening is essential to the communication process.

- Ideas cannot be transferred directly from one person to another. Mental filters and perceived meaning often produce static in the communication process. To the listener, total meaning is a mixture of intellectual and emotional associations. That is why communication experts have paid so much attention to body language—the facial expressions, gestures, and inflections that can make or break communications.

- Words do not have meaning within themselves. All of us derive meaning from experience, and therefore words have different meanings for different people.

- Meanings, attitudes, beliefs, and expectancies, once established, tend to remain stable. Present meanings, attitudes, and expectancies tend to be unconsciously supported and reinforced.

- Because of already established attitudes and expectancies, certain methods of communication and certain communicators may be rejected. There is no question that much of such rejection is emotional.[4]

FEEDBACK

Because it is difficult to convey meaning, and because the full meaning of any message is affected by the total personality and experience of the employee receiving the message, feedback is important. Simply stated, you do not really know what you have communicated until you have received feedback. Feedback should be considered a way of giving help. It is essential information supplied by others to help people discover their effectiveness as communicators. Feedback can be either corrective or confirming; an employee needs both. With a continual flow of reliable feedback, supervisors can determine whether they are "on target" and can make any necessary changes.

Feedback can tell the receivers how their behavior appears to others or affects the feelings of others. Each individual is free to use or not use the feedback.

Feedback is not evaluative. It is focused on specific behavior, not on the quality of the person. By avoiding personal evaluation, there is no need for the individual to act defensively. Each person's perception of other people is somewhat distorted. Therefore, feedback from one person should always be checked against feedback from others.

A little feedback is better than none at all, but the more feedback the better. The supervisor should not limit the employee to simple yes or no responses but rather encourage open responses and questions.

LISTENING—THE LOST ART

If there is one area where many modern supervisors fail, it is in communication. Communication is the best way to reach agreement on an institution's objectives and to direct efforts toward meeting those objectives. In an American Management Association study of superior-subordinate communication at the managerial level, researchers found:

> If a *single* answer can be drawn from this detailed study into superior-subordinate communication on the managerial level, . . . it is this: If one is speaking of the subordinate's specific job—his duties, the requirements he must fulfill in order to do his work well, his intelligent anticipation of future changes in his work, and the obstacles which prevent him from doing as good a job as possible—he and his boss do not agree, in almost every area. . . . [5]

Over the years, convincing evidence has emerged to prove that we waste energy and economic resources by concentrating on the *form* of communication rather than its *substance*. Many people have the counterproductive habit of seeking driving directions at gas stations or from a pedestrian or other driver and then riding away without having absorbed the instructions. *They did not listen.* Half the process of communication is listening—not just sitting back and hearing, but listening. There is a distinct difference between hearing and listening. Hearing denotes an awareness of the transmission of sound. Listening denotes an ability to understand, comprehend, and retain what has been said.

The cliché, "What we have here is a failure to communicate," can be paraphrased, "What we have here is the result of poor listening habits." The better listeners supervisors are, the better listeners they will inspire. If you listen to people, your chances increase that they will listen to you. If you fail to listen to people, the chances are slim that they will listen to you. Normally, one kind of behavior brings about a like behavior.

GAINING COOPERATION IS HALF THE BATTLE

More often than not, change requires cooperation. There are few instances of a single individual developing and implementing a specific change. The need for cooperation is underscored. If there is an area of supervisory skill that should be honed to perfection, it is the supervisor's responsibility to gain cooperation to ensure a smooth and expeditious transition from the old to the new.

One expert suggests that the following skills, when applied, can create a spirit of effective teamwork:

Avoid arguments. Understand what the other person is concerned about and listen beyond the emotions. This, of course, requires letting the other person tell the full story without interruption. Criticism should be minimized. Criticizing your subordinate may win you the battle, but you will certainly lose the war. The key to gaining agreement is to move from small points of consensus to overall and final agreement on the totality of the change.

Admit your errors. We are all vulnerable; very few of us can state that we are never wrong. It is well to remember that people do not like others who are "always right." Admitting your mistakes when they are made will gain you immeasurable respect from your subordinates.

Establish a receptive frame of mind. This can be accomplished by explaining why the change has to be implemented and how it will benefit all—yourself and your subordinates. Emphasize the need for cooperation and the essential role the subordinate plays in implementing the change. Ask for ideas and suggestions on moving from present methods to new methods. Receptivity seldom comes by fiat—you cannot legislate a receptive frame of mind. The supervisor's task is to develop conditions that will encourage the subordinate to listen and be objective. Once you have established this receptive frame of mind you can rest assured your subordinates will be cooperative.

A sympathetic "no" is better than a harsh "yes." Gaining agreement at any price is poor supervisory practice. You will have to say no at times. More often than not, if the no is said in a sympathetic and understanding way, it will not produce negative reactions. Use a friendly, nonthreatening approach; show a sincere interest in the reactions of your employees; explain the reasons for your no; and, finally, express your appreciation.

Dramatize ideas or suggestions. Of all the senses, that of sight is the strongest. Therefore, it is most helpful to dramatize the ideas or suggestions for change by use of visual aids—including diagrams, charts, and films.

Set a fair challenge. Your employees will normally rise to challenges. A great deal of research has indicated that employees perform better and are more cooperative when they are presented with a challenging goal.

Praise in advance. The need for appreciation stands at the top of the pyramid of employee wants. In the very complicated and hierarchical structures of most health care facilities, employees at the bottom rung often feel like invisible people. Praise should not be bestowed grudgingly. Given the highly important work in health care facilities and the day-to-day pressures, praise is vital. Supervisors may reply, "There just isn't enough time," but the successful supervisor is able to find something to commend in even the least competent person.

Don't demand cooperation. It just is not possible to force people to cooperate. At most, you will get surface cooperation. True cooperation can come only on a voluntary basis.[6]

RESEARCH STUDIES ON WORKER PARTICIPATION IN MANAGEMENT

There is more and more evidence that when workers are allowed to make some decisions about their own work, they will be more productive. Most of the plans to increase worker participation attempt to develop a spirit of cooperation and teamwork on the job. The same principle can be applied to the facilitating of change. One research study found that where subordinates are allowed to express themselves and decision making is shared between the supervisor and the subordinate—decision making by consensus rather than by fiat—there is a marked reduction in rivalry and conflict and a greater sense of psychological success. Decisions reached by consensus have enormous positive effects on productivity. When subordinates have a voice in significant problem-solving activities and therefore more responsibility for their own and their fellow workers' futures, they often experience a greater sense of interdependence between themselves and the whole, an enlarged awareness of the whole, a better time perspective, and a greater capacity to change the organization's internal makeup. The same study cautions that, unless the participants truly believe and behave in ways consistent with these new values, the "changes suggested . . . will fail because they will be perceived by the subordinates for what they really are: gimmicks and techniques to manipulate people and . . . place power in the hands of people who do not tend to trust one another or probably themselves."[7]

Research has been done on the features of the hospital management structure that lead to alienation of nonsupervisory personnel. In particular, this research has tested the hypothesis that the degree of alienation is related to the degree to which nonsupervisory nursing personnel are allowed to participate in a management decision. The results indicated that alienation is greater in situations where nonsupervisory staff are not allowed to participate in the decision-making process and that inflexible bureaucratic systems tend to cause frustrations and depersonalization of staff relations, causing loss of initiative.[8]

The supervisor should encourage subordinates' participation in establishing criteria for group and individual performance. In this way, subordinates help determine the basis on which their efforts will be judged. Just as important, this involves subordinates in the planning process, which increases their commitment to the agreed-upon goals and objectives.

Coch and French conducted a study on overcoming resistance to change in a factory. There were three groups in the study. Group 1 was the control group. Group 2 featured participation by representatives of the workers in designing job changes. Group 3 featured total participation by all members of the group.

In Group 1, the control group, the production department modified the job, set the new piece rate, and then held a group meeting to communicate the change. Workers were told that the change was necessary because of competitive conditions, and the new piece rate was explained by the time-study man. Questions were answered. The results were disappointing: the group decreased production, a result related to the workers' overall rejection of a change they saw as arbitrary and unreasonable.

In Group 2, the plant manager met with representatives of the group and there was joint planning. Again the competitive picture was emphasized. The representatives were exposed to a dramatic presentation of the change. Two identical garments were displayed. Members of the group were asked to identify the cheaper one, and they could not. Yet one of the garments was produced the year before and the other was new. It was clearly and dramatically explained that the new garment was the cheaper one. The management then presented its plan for change and the new piece rate. The representatives were informed of the need to eliminate all unnecessary work. Several operators were trained in the new methods, and a piece rate agreeable to the representatives of the group was set. The results? Within two weeks productivity was satisfactory and met the competitive needs.

In Group 3, the plant manager met with individual workers. The methods used in Group 2 were used, but here every worker participated. *Every worker was involved in meetings and every worker was consulted.* In a matter of days, this group reached peak efficiency. These findings suggest that broad participation and planning for change reduce resistance dramatically.[9]

THE TALKING CHIEFS

Merrihue starts his book on communications with an apocryphal story:

> Ganduki was a newly chosen warrior chieftain of an African tribe in a remote vastness in the vast Belgian Congo. Much irked by the poaching and sporadic raids of a persistent chief in a rival tribe, Ganduki called together his warriors and after a six day march, liquidated the troublesome tribe in a brilliant coup distinguished by its strategy and his personal courage. On the long trek home, Ganduki was sorely troubled despite the great victory and the booty

and the slaves his warriors were bringing back. A man of action, but inarticulate, he would rather wage another battle than face up to the victory speech his tribe would expect upon his return. So calling upon his medicine man, Bo-Gobi, he prevailed upon him to communicate the magnitude and the brilliance of the victory to the homefolks.

And so it was. After hours of feasting, Bo-Gobi mounted an ivory dais and began the narrative of the battle. As he warmed to his task to the rising crescendo of the throbbing drums, the gaudily painted, spearwaving warriors leaped and howled in the eerie light cast by the roaring fire and when he had completed his tale, Bo-Gobi was caught up in the arms of his tribesmen and with a mighty shout, they hailed him as their savior and newly elected chief.[10]

Clear enough? The chiefs who master the ability to talk—to communicate—are accepted as true leaders. Your skill as a communicator is essential to your success as a supervisor and to the productivity of your work crew. No matter how varied your activities may be and how specialized your skills are, in the final analysis your success as a supervisor is related to communication. In short, the supervisor gets work done through other people; to accomplish this the supervisor must communicate effectively.

You must be especially careful about upward communication. Your subordinates often tell you what they think you want to hear. They will minimize incidents that will result in your vindictiveness or unhappiness. If you want to obtain accurate information, you must develop an organizational style based on trust and confidence—one that invites a free flow and exchange of information up and down the line. You cannot assume that subordinates share your contentment and satisfaction with the organization. Too often people tend to hear what they want to hear and to close their ears to what they do not want to hear. If you are to obtain honest and objective communication from your subordinates, they have got to believe that you are operating with honesty and objectivity. Has what you've told them in the past been accurate, open, and factual? Can they rely on your word?

You never communicate in a vacuum. Effective communication flows from sound employee relations. If your subordinates believe that you do not play favorites, that you do not take all the credit, that you do not pass the buck, that you do back them up, that you are fair and dependable, they will listen to what you have to say.

HOW TO PRODUCE MORE EFFECTIVE COMMUNICATION

Merrihue suggests that if you as a first-line supervisor hope to meet the universal standards for effective communication with your employees, you will first need to gain the confidence of your employees by

- being impartial and consistent,
- making no commitments that you cannot fulfill,
- making certain that all problems and grievances are answered promptly and correctly,
- making the employees' work problems your own, and actively representing your employees' interests to other levels of management, and
- making it clear that the institution has grievance machinery that works.

Second, you must gain the respect and friendship of your employees by

- according respectful treatment to each employee as an individual and esteemed associate, showing sincere interest in that employee's welfare,
- displaying enthusiasm over the employees' progress,
- being considerate and helpful in all possible ways,
- demonstrating your sincere personal interest in matters that are important to them—by attending weddings and funerals, delivering pay and benefit checks in person when employees are ill, attending social affairs and family nights together, and so on.

Third, having established the proper climate for good downward communication to receptive employees and good upward communication from employees who feel free to discuss matters with you, you will need to develop your skills in (1) listening, (2) talking, and (3) selling. Of these skills, none is more important than the ability to listen carefully in order to achieve full understanding of the information received, to take action quickly based on this understanding, and to communicate the results of such action to the individuals involved.[11]

It is suggested that you ask yourself these six questions before you attempt to communicate to your employees:

1. Do I assume that if an idea is clear to me it will be clear to the receiver? (Just not so!)
2. Do I make it comfortable for others to tell me what is really on their minds—or do I encourage them to tell me only what I would like to hear? (It had better be the former!)
3. Do I check my understanding of what another person has told me before I reply? (Feedback is essential to effective communication!)
4. Am I tolerant of other people's feelings, realizing that their feelings, which may be different from mine, affect their communication? (We are always dealing with human emotions!)
5. Do I really try to listen from the sender's point of view before evaluating the message from my point of view? (There are two people in most conversations; the other person has a point of view!)
6. Do I make a conscious effort to build a feedback mechanism into all communications, in view of the fact that, even at its best, communication is an imperfect process? (Did the other person hear what I meant to say?)

With the advent of large institutions and complex delivery systems, the modern supervisor is equipped with techniques and methods far superior to those previously available. But we have all paid a high price for this specialization. Indeed, in an era of overspecialization, we as supervisors are no longer directly involved; in contrast with our earlier counterpart and present-day workers, we must get the job done through others. Only to the extent that we develop and refine the art of communication, we will be effective supervisors.

PRINCIPLES OF EFFECTIVE COMMUNICATION

We communicate in many ways: orally, in face-to-face-communications with our employees; by memorandum; through bulletins on bulletin boards; and in meetings—in conferences and lectures, with or without group participation. There is no question that successful organizations are successful in the area of communications. No matter what form communication takes, there is a sender and there is a receiver. The sender needs a receiver who will tune in to the message and clear up the static. Here are some underlying principles for effective employee-supervisor communication:

- Communication should not be regarded as a tool or a *helping* aspect of the organization but rather as the essence of organized activity and the basic process from which all other functions derive.

- Communication should be subject to the same controls as other organizational activities—that is, the accepted management principles of analysis planning, coordination, and evaluation.

- Communication should be thought of as directional—upward, downward, or horizontal from the sender.

- Ineffective communication can mean wasted time and resources and, therefore, can result in lower productivity and higher costs.

- We communicate in a variety of ways, verbal and nonverbal (through gestures, facial expressions, body postures and movements, tone of voice, and dress). Most of all, we communicate by our actions.

- People will generally hear, read, observe, and choose to understand only those parts of a message that relate to their own interests, desires, and needs.

- One cannot *not* communicate. When a response is expected and is not forthcoming, silence communicates fear, stubbornness, uncooperativeness, and so on. Thus, our choice is not between communicating and not communicating, but between communicating effectively and communicating ineffectively, between contributing or not contributing to organizational goals.

- Although many supervisors feel that a message need be transmitted only once, specialists insist that repetition is important.

- Communication is generally more effective when it provides the means for *feedback*. Without feedback the sender cannot know what effect the message has had on the receiver's behavior, nor can the sender know how to achieve better communication next time. Communications that provide for feedback are called *two-way communications.*

- Although effective communication requires an expert use of media, the greatest barrier to communication probably lies in the area of human relations. Communication does not occur merely because a message is sent; it must also be received with reasonable fidelity.[12]

The following is a list of seven key points on how to communicate changes:

1. As a supervisor you must initiate changes at a faster rate than ever before.
2. Most employees react to change with resistance. You should understand that resistance and work with it.
3. To minimize resistance, you should explain in advance the need for change, gain consensus, and establish a receptive frame of mind.
4. You must not personalize the change. You should indicate clearly and dramatically how the change will benefit the individual and the group.
5. You should effect a feedback loop. Make sure that you are on target. Remember that what you *mean* to say is not always what you *actually* say or what the other person *hears*. Feedback is a method of establishing understanding. It is a mirror, not a directive. Feedback is possible only when subordinates believe they can be frank and honest.
6. Half the process of communication is listening. The better listeners supervisors are, the better listening they will inspire.
7. People who participate in the shaping of change are more likely to be receptive to the change and, therefore, more productive. Increased participation in decision making can be an effective management tool, depending on the management style that has preceded it. If your subordinates believe that you truly value their ideas, that you will consider their suggestions objectively, that they can be free to voice their concerns to you—then and only then will participation be effective.

COMMUNICATING CHANGE REVIEW PUZZLE

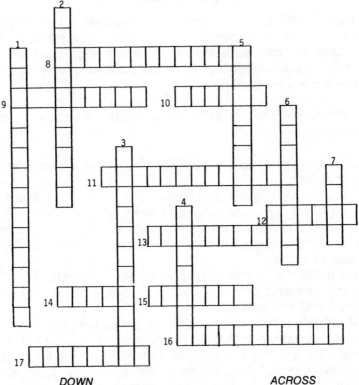

DOWN

1) A prophecy that can determine the outcome of change.
2) Reinforces the retention of messages.
3) To obtain change you must have this.
4) These behaviors communicate.
5) What feedback should *not* be.
6) Communication flow that is typical of most institutions.
7) First impressions are normally formed in the first _____minutes.

ACROSS

8) What decision making should be.
9) The lost "art."
10) What communication should be (two words).
11) Essential to good employee relations.
12) You never communicate in a _____.
13) Messages must be _____.
14) Supervisory style must be based on this.
15) Communication should be thought of as a _____.
16) They play a key role as agents of change.
17) A requirement of change.

(Answers are on page 21.)

NOTES

1. Willard V. Merrihue, *Managing by Communication* (New York: McGraw-Hill Company, 1960), p. 243.
2. Leo B. Moore, "Too Much Management, Too Little Change," *Harvard Business Review*, January-February, 1956, p. 41.
3. W.G. Bennis, K.D. Benne, and R. Chin, *The Planning of Change* (New York: Holt, Rhinehart, and Winston, 1964), passim.
4. P. Ecker et al., *Handbook for Supervisors* (Englewood Cliffs, N.J.: Prentice Hall, Inc., 1959), pp. 167-169.
5. N.R.S. Maier et al., *Superior-Subordinate Communication in Management, Report No. 52*. (New York: American Management Association, 1961), p. 9.
6. Alfred R. Lateiner, *Modern Techniques of Supervision* (Stamford, Conn.: Lateiner Publishing Co.) or Alfred R. Lateiner, *The Technique of Supervision* (New London, Conn.: National Fireman's Institute, 1954), pp. 28-29.
7. Chris Agyris, *The Integration of the Individual in the Organization—Social Science Approaches to Business Behavior* (Homewood, Ill.: Dorsey Press, 1962), pp. 85-87.
8. Jeanne LaPorte, "Participatory Management—The Technique to Alleviate Alienation of Bureaucratic Organizations, thesis, University of Ottawa, Ontario, May 1972, passim.
9. L. Coch and J.R.P. French, "Overcoming Resistance to Change," in Dorwin Cartwright and Alvin Zander, eds., *Group Dynamics: Research and Theory*, 2nd ed. (Evanston, Ill.: Row Peterson and Company, 1960), passim.
10. Merrihue, *Managing by Communication*, p. 1.
11. Ibid., pp. 108-109.
12. Training Research and Special Studies Division, United Hospital Fund, *Improving Employee Management Communication in Hospitals, A Special Study in Management Practices and Problems* (New York: Training Research and Special Studies Division, United Hospital Fund, 1965), pp. 10-11.

SUGGESTED READINGS

Barnlund, Dean C. "Communication in the Context of Change." In *Perspectives on Communication*, edited by C.E. Larson and F.E.X. Dance. Milwaukee: University of Wisconsin Communication Research Center, 1968, pp. 25-41.

Bennis, Warren; Benne, K.D.; and Chin, R. *The Planning of Change*. New York: Holt, Rhinehart, and Winston, 1964.

———; Schien, Edgar; Steele, Fred; and Berlew, David. "Personal Change Through Interpersonal Relationships." In *Interpersonal Dynamics: Essays and Readings on Human Interaction*, edited by Warren Bennis and Edgar Schien. Homewood, Ill.: Dorsey Press, 1968, pp. 333-369.

Buchanan, Paul C. "How Can We Gain Their Commitment?" *Personnel* 42(1965): 21-26.

Coch, L., and French, J.R.P. "Overcoming Resistance to Change." In *Group Dynamics: Research and Theory*, edited by Dorwin Cartwright and Alvin Zander. Evanston, Ill.: Row Peterson and Company, 1960, pp. 336-350.

Cohen, A. *Attitude Change and Social Influence*. New York: Basic Books, 1964.

Griener, Larry. "Patterns of Organization Change." *Harvard Business Review* 45(1967): 119-130.

Hain, Tony. *Patterns of Organizational Change*. Flint, Mich.: General Motors Institute, 1972.

Insko, Chester. *Theories of Attitude Change*. New York: Appleton-Century-Crofts, 1967.

Leavitt, Harold J. "Applied Organizational Change in Industry: Structural, Technological, and Humanistic Approaches." In *Handbook of Organizations*, edited by J.G. March. Chicago: Rand McNally, 1965, pp. 1144-1170.

Marrow, A.J.; Bowers, D.G.; and Seashore, S.E.; eds. *Organizational Change*. New York: Harper & Row, 1967.

Schien, Edgar, and Bennis, Warren. *Personal and Organizational Change*. New York: Wiley and Sons, 1965.

Sherif, Muzafer, and Sherif, Carolyn. *Attitude Ego-involvement and Change*. New York: John Wiley, 1967.

Triandis, Harry C. *Attitude and Attitude Change*. New York: John Wiley, 1971.

Zimbardo, P., and Ebbesen, E.B. *Influencing Attitudes and Changing Behavior*. Reading, Mass.: Addison-Wesley, 1969.

COMMUNICATING CHANGE REVIEW PUZZLE

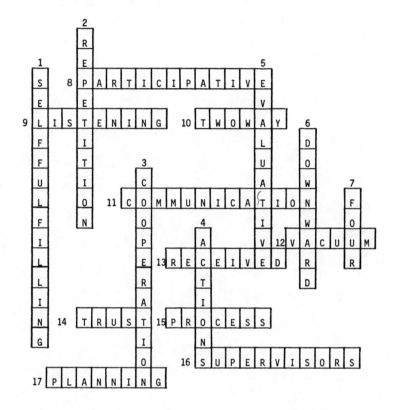

DOWN

1) A prophecy that can determine the outcome of change.
2) Reinforces the retention of messages.
3) To obtain change you must have this.
4) These behaviors communicate.
5) What feedback should *not* be.
6) Communication flow that is typical of most institutions.
7) First impressions are normally formed in the first ____minutes.

ACROSS

8) What decision making should be.
9) The lost "art."
10) What communication should be (two words).
11) Essential to good employee relations.
12) You never communicate in a ____.
13) Messages must be ____.
14) Supervisory style must be based on this.
15) Communication should be thought of as a ____.
16) They play a key role as agents of change.
17) A requirement of change.

Chapter 2

The Supervisor As an Organizational Climate Maker

CHAPTER OBJECTIVES

The purpose of this chapter is to enable you to CHANGE your communicative behavior in a *positive* direction. After studying the material you should be able to:

Comprehend the importance of organizational climate.

Help your work group improve its organizational climate.

Analyze the existing organizational climate in your work group.

Notice the effects of organizational climate on patients, coworkers, and employees.

Guide your work group toward greater group cohesion.

Examine your role as a climate maker.

INTRODUCTION

What is organizational climate? Can it be used to motivate and enhance the performance of workers? The dimensions of an organizational climate seem to vary from theorist to theorist, but the combined research seems to suggest that various small-group variables determine the organizational climate of a group.

William Evans has defined organizational climate as "a multidimensional perception by members, as well as nonmembers, of the essential attributes or character of an organizational system."[1]

There are certain properties that may be classified as attributes that help form the character of an organization. These attributes or properties play an instrumental role in developing group climate.

Dorwin Cartwright has identified nine group properties that appear to have potential value, depending upon the motives of the people involved:

1. attractiveness of group members
2. similarities among members
3. nature of group goals
4. type of interdependence among group members
5. activities of the group
6. style of leadership and the opportunity to participate in decisions
7. various structural properties of the group
8. the group atmosphere
9. size of the group[2]

Evans makes the following assumptions about organizational climate:

- Members as well as nonmembers have perceptions about the climate of the organization.

- Organizational members tend to perceive the climate differently from nonmembers because of the prevalence of different frames of reference and different criteria for evaluating the organization.

- Perceptions of organizational climate, whether real or unreal, have behavioral consequences for the organization as well as for the organization-set, i.e., the complement of organizations with which the organization interacts.

- Organizational members performing differing roles tend to have different perceptions of the climate, if only because of (1) a lack of role census, (2) a lack of uniformity in role socialization, (3) a diversity in patterns of role-set interactions.

- Members of different organizational subunits tend to have different perceptions of the climate because of different role-set configurations, different subgoals, and different subcommitments to the goals of subunits compared to the goals of the organization as a whole.[3]

As further clarification, Andrew Halpin offers the following metaphorical description of organizational climate:

> Anyone who visits more than a few schools notes quickly how schools differ from each other in their "feel." In one school the teacher and students are zestful and exude confidence in what they are doing. They find pleasure in working with each other; this pleasure is transmitted to the students, who thus are given at least a fighting chance to discover that the school can be a happy experience. In a second school the brooding discontent of the teachers is palpable; the principal tries to hide his incompetence and his lack of sense of direction behind a cloak of authority, and yet he wears his cloak poorly because the attitude he displays toward others vacillates randomly between the obsequious and the officious. And the psychological sickness of such a faculty spills over on the students who, in their own frustration, feed back to the teachers a mood of despair. A third school is neither marked by joy nor despair, but by hollow ritual. Here one gets the feeling of watching an elaborate charade in which teachers, principal and students are acting out parts. The acting is smooth, even glib, but it appears to have little meaning for the participants; in a strange way the show just doesn't seem to be "for real." And so, too, as one moves to other schools, one finds that each appears to have a "personality" of its own. It is this personality that we describe here as organizational climate of the school.[4]

We could easily substitute hospital, clinic, nursing home, or any other type of health care facility for school in the preceding metaphorical description of organizational climate. In fact, you could walk through your own facility and find unique, but obvious, differences in the organizational climate of subgroups.

THE HEALTH CARE ORGANIZATIONAL CLIMATE

What is organizational climate in a health care setting? This can be answered best in terms of an analogy. Organizational climate is both similar to and different from the weather. For example, more than 20 percent of the American population watches the weather report each night to find out what the weather will be like the next day. In another context, the climate affects our relationships with people. Doesn't the behavior of people toward one another seem to be different on a clear, bright, 70-degree Spring day compared to a stormy, 10-degree day with sleet and snow?

Considerable evidence seems to indicate that, just as people tend to take cues on clothing and behavior from the weather, they are also influenced by the kind of organizational climate within their organization. Thus, the organizational climate within a hospital will affect the behavior of supervisors, employees, doctors, nurses, technicians, aides, and patients.

At this point, however, the analogy ends, and the differences between the weather and organizational climate begin to appear. Unlike the weather, the organizational climate of a hospital is not something that we can directly see or touch. We can nevertheless sense it just as easily as a nurse or physician can sense that something is wrong with a patient. Though no thermometer can measure it, the organizational climate can be manipulated and changed. The real weather of wind, rain, and snow cannot be changed and goes its merry way. But people create their own work environment; if it isn't right, people can change it.

Numerous studies have shown that certain types of climates typify high performance groups. The recent move back to primary nursing and the decentralization within hospitals indicate that climate making can influence how employees feel about their work. The resulting feelings are then transmitted into hard realities, such as individual motivation and effort, goal clarity, group cohesiveness, and a continuing commitment to goals.

No matter how many positive factors—such as good planning by supervisors and health care knowledge—there are within a hospital, many of the pitfalls encountered by the hospital in getting the job done will involve human problems, and such problems relate to bottom line performance, that is, excellent patient care.

The behavior a supervisor exhibits on the job helps to determine the organizational climate. The combined human behaviors of all health care employees determine the total organizational climate of the hospital. By exhibiting "positive" communicative behaviors supervisors can:

- make their work group more cohesive,

- help others to motivate themselves,

- improve the organizational climate, and

- create a balance between the pressures for high short-term performance and the development of individual talents of the people they work with.

K.W. Back discovered that highly cohesive groups tended to place more value on communication than groups of low cohesion. The highly cohesive groups also had more communicative balance among their members. No one member seemed to dominate the thinking of the group.[5]

DIMENSIONS OF CLIMATE

There are six climate dimensions that can be categorized into two groups: (1) performance dimensions and (2) development dimensions. Through an understanding of these dimensions of climate and by applying them to their jobs, supervisors can increase their effectiveness as motivational agents.

Performance Dimensions

Clarity

Clarity refers to the supervisor's sense of understanding of the hospital's goals and policies. This requires an effort to make things run smoothly, as opposed to an acceptance of confusion. Supervisors will change the organizational climate in a positive direction if

- they help their employees to understand what is expected of them,

- they help their employees plan and organize activities, and
- they see that information flows smoothly.

Commitment

Supervisors must have a continuing commitment to goal achievement. This commitment is related to acceptance of realistic goals, an involvement in goal setting, and a continuous evaluation of performance compared to goals. Supervisors will change the organizational climate in a positive direction if

- they involve their employees in goal setting and review meetings,
- their employees recognize the goals and consider them to be meaningful and realistic, and
- their employees have a personal commitment to achieve the goals.

Cartwright has stated that "the greater the group's cohesion the more power it has to bring about conformity to its norms and to gain acceptance of its goals and assignments to tasks and roles."[6]

Standards

Here the focus is on the emphasis that the supervisor places on setting high standards of performance. Supervisors will change the organizational climate in a positive direction if

- they are interested in improving individual performance,
- they can instill pride in doing a job well, and
- they set tough and challenging personal goals.

Alvin Zander has found that a group's aspiration level helped to determine its degree of success or failure.

> After repeated success, members who perceive that the future promises a greater likelihood of success at that level of difficulty, raise their anticipated level of aspiration, develop feelings of success and pride in the group, assign a favorable evaluation to their group's performance, attri-

bute greater value to future success, develop a disposition to seek further success, perceive their group to be an attractive one, and become committed to the process of setting future goals. Individuals who have more responsible positions are more likely to have the reactions just described than are those with less important roles.

On the other hand, after repeated failure, members are less inclined to be concerned about the probabilities of future failure, or success; instead, they seek means that will help them avoid the unfavorable consequences of failure. They tend to: lower the group's goal or stick with the one they have failed to reach, give an unapproving evaluation to their group's performance, see the activity as less important, believe that success on the task is less desirable, are less attracted to their own group, and would like to judge the group in relation to its past performance rather than its goal attainment. They would gladly abandon altogether the practice of setting aspiration levels. Members of such groups have a distinct preference for unreasonably difficult tasks, in the light of their past performance, making them highly vulnerable to subsequent failure.[7]

Development Dimensions

Responsibility

This dimension concerns the supervisor's feelings of personal responsibility for work, involving both a sense of autonomy stemming from real delegation and encouragement to take individual initiatives. Supervisors will change the organizational climate in a positive direction if

- they feel they can help employees solve problems,
- they help employees to develop a sense of independence and to feel that the employees' judgment is trusted, and
- they encourage themselves and their employees to take increased responsibility.

Cartwright discovered that members of cohesive groups more readily exert influence over one another and are more readily influenced by one another, compared to members of noncohesive groups.[8]

Recognition

Supervisors must feel that they and their employees will be recognized for doing a good job. They should not feel that criticism is more likely than recognition for good performance. Supervisors will change the organizational climate in a positive direction if

- they help their employees to see that rewards and recognition outweigh threats and criticism,

- their employees see the existence of a promotion system that helps the best person rise to the top, and

- their employees see rewards related to excellence of performance.

J.W. Thibaut and H.H. Kelley discovered that a person will join a group based on personal expected outcomes.

> When joining a group a person employs a standard called the comparison level, against which they compare the expected outcomes of membership. This comparison level derives from their previous experience in groups and indicates the level of outcomes they aspire to receive from membership. They will be more attracted to the group the more the level of expected outcomes exceeds their comparison level.[9]

Teamwork

Hospital supervisors and employees must feel that they belong to a health care team. This feeling is characterized by cohesion, mutual warmth, support, trust, and pride. Supervisors will change the organizational climate in a positive direction if

- they help their employees to see mutual understanding and support,

- their employees see people trusting and respecting others, and

- they help their employees to develop a feeling of personal loyalty and a sense of belonging to their work group.

Rensis Likert found that group morale and team spirit increased when

> The leadership and other processes of the organization ensure a maximum probability that in all interactions and in all relationships with the organization members will, in the light of their background, values, and expectations, view the experience as supportive and one which builds and maintains their sense of personal worth and importance.[10]

The key to Likert's conclusion is in the role of trust. High trust tends to stimulate high performance and increased employee confidence, loyalty, and teamwork.[11]

A CLIMATE OF DISBELIEF

Harish Jain, in his doctoral dissertation, collected questionnaire-type data from both superiors and subordinates in two hospitals, designated Hospital X and Hospital Y. He was investigating possible relationships between a set of communicative variables and a set of supervisory effectiveness variables. Hospital X contained 721 beds and 1700 employees. Hospital Y had 200 beds and 500 employees. In Hospital X he obtained the questionnaire data from 122 employees and 8 management personnel. In Hospital Y he obtained the same type of data from 90 employees and 8 management personnel. In addition, he interviewed in depth 45 nonsupervisory workers who formed a subsample of respondents.

The research hypotheses were: (1) The higher the score on supervisory communication attitudes, the more favorable will be the supervisory effectiveness ratings. (2) The greater the communication satisfaction of employees, the more favorable will be the supervisory effectiveness ratings.[12]

Supervisory effectiveness was defined in three categories: human relations, administrative skills, and technical skills. In general, both hypotheses were supported by the collected data. In Hospital X, however, the ratings from "technical workers" did not corroborate the predicted relationships. The research uncovered a number of sources of discontent, extending from oppressive regulations on punctuality to lack of leadership and favoritism on the part of supervisors.[13]

Jain then interviewed the technical employees at Hospital X. He discovered that there were other mediating variables, not directly measured in his study, that were responsible for the lack of relationship between communication and supervisory effectiveness:

> . . . one such variable was a *climate of disbelief* which permeated the department. . . . in order for communication to be effective between his supervisor and subordinates, or any other level in the organization, it must be preceded by a climate of belief. The only way a climate of belief could be brought about was by building employee confidence and trust in leadership. In other words, the leaders . . . had to share information with their subordinates, consult them on matters of mutual interest and settle their grievances promptly. None of these ingredients seemed to be present in the department . . . of Hospital X. The technicians had no trust in the leaders of their units.[14]

The technicians in Hospital Y, on the other hand, worked in close proximity and had the opportunity to communicate with one another. They also revealed a high degree of trust in their supervisors. In Hospital Y, the variables of communicative attitude, communicative satisfaction, and supervisory effectiveness were found to be positively correlated in both hypotheses. The group in Hospital Y apparently indulged in a great deal of face-to-face communication between subordinates and supervisors.[15]

The decision to spend time improving the organizational climate within a hospital work group is one that supervisors must make for themselves. Each supervisor has the responsibility to encourage others in individual or joint efforts. Highly motivated individuals tend to work in supportive organizational climates. But it should be remembered that people make the climate. We live in climates of our own making, and these self-made climates affect our relationships with others.

A supportive climate extends into every hospital unit. No one can see it or touch it, but every health care employee and patient can sense it. When employees sense a supportive organizational climate, it reaffirms their basic reason for being, for caring about people and improved patient care.

A SUPERVISORY CLIMATE SURVEY

The following supervisory climate survey is aimed at gaining a better understanding of the kind of work climate or environment in which your employees work, of the way in which the climate is created, and how it affects job performance and ultimately the job satisfaction of the employee.

As you fill out the questionnaire, respond to the items as they relate to your work group. Do not assume that pay, money, or economic gains are implied by any of the questions. That is, questions that deal with recognition assume nonfinancial recognition.

PART I

For each of the statements below please draw a circle around one of the following:

A—Always
F—Frequently
O—Occasionally
S—Seldom
N—Never

For example, if you feel that you are frequently encouraged to come up with new and original ideas, you would circle the "F" in the following question:

A Ⓕ O S N   1. We are encouraged to come up with new and original ideas.

Please use only one evaluative letter code for each answer.

A F O S N   1. I have the opportunity to review my overall performance and effectiveness with my supervisor.

A F O S N   2. There is much respect between management and other personnel in this group.

A F O S N   3. In this organization, the rewards and encouragements you receive for effective performance outweigh the threats and criticisms.

A F O S N   4. Our people are encouraged to make decisions when the situation demands an immediate decision.

A F O S N   5. In this group, I am given a chance to participate in setting the performance goals for my job.

A F O S N   6. People in our group are aware of what good performance means in their jobs.

A F O S N   7. I feel that I am a member of a well-functioning team.

A F O S N   8. In this group we are rewarded in proportion to how well we do our jobs.

A F O S N   9. We are encouraged to come up with new and original ideas.

A F O S N   10. Management works with us in developing challenging team and group goals.

A F O S N   11. In this group, performance is evaluated against agreed-upon performance goals.

A F O S N   12. In my group, high performers are recognized by their supervisor for their superior performance.

A F O S N   13. In this group, what constitutes good performance has been identified.

A F O S N   14. In this group, people demonstrate strong commitment to achieving performance goals.

A F O S N   15. Things seem to be fairly well organized in my group.

A F O S N   16. People in this group help each other in solving job-related problems.

A F O S N   17. My supervisor does a good job in recognizing good performance.

A F O S N   18. My supervisor emphasizes that people in this group should personally accept the responsibility for solving day-to-day operational problems.

A F O S N   19. In this group, we are encouraged to improve continually our personal and group performance.

A F O S N   20. The results I am supposed to achieve in my job are realistic.

A F O S N   21. The policies and structure of this group have been clearly explained.

A F O S N   22. People are proud to belong to this group.

A F O S N   23. In my group, very high standards are set for performance.

A F O S N   24. I am involved in setting my own performance goals and in understanding how they relate to the overall goals of my group.

A F O S N   25. The assignments in my group are clearly defined and logically structured.

If your responses were in the "always" or "frequently" columns, you see your work group in a very positive way. On the other hand, if most of your responses were "seldom" or "never," you see your group in a very negative way, and this can affect your morale.

Working conditions and an employee's perceptions of those conditions affect individual morale and determine the work climate. If the organizational climate of a hospital is not right, can an employee change that climate? Can an employee become a motivational agent of change? Remember, organizational climate does not just happen. Rather it is the "collective" view of the people within an organization as to the nature of the environment in which they work, and they can make that climate anything they want it to be.

CLIMATE REVIEW PUZZLE

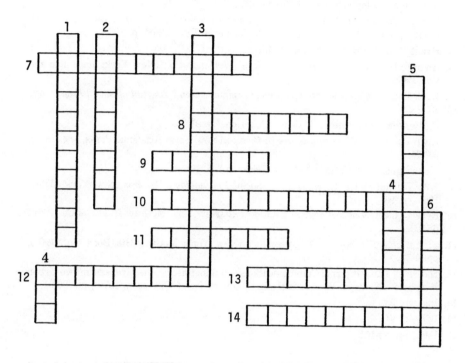

DOWN

1) A major climate dimension.
2) Determines organizational climate.
3) Affected by organizational climate.
4) Number of performance dimensions.
5) A performance dimension.
6) Similar to but different from organizational climate.

ACROSS

7) A major climate dimension.
8) A development dimension.
9) Who creates organizational climate?
10) A development dimension.
11) A collective organizational view.
12) A performance dimension.
13) Another performance dimension.
14) Highly motivated individuals tend to work in _____ organizational climates.

(Answers are on page 40.)

NOTES

1. William Evans, *Organizational Theory: Structures, Systems, and Environment* (New York: John Wiley and Sons, 1976), p. 137.
2. Dorwin Cartwright, "The Nature of Group Cohesion," in *Group Dynamics*, ed. D. Cartwright and A. Zander (New York: Harper & Row, 1968), p. 107.
3. Evans, *Organizational Theory*, p. 139.
4. Andrew Halpin, *Theory and Research in Administration* (New York: Macmillan and Co., 1966), p. 131.
5. K.W. Back, "Influence Through Social Communication," *Journal of Social Psychology* 46: 9-23.
6. Cartwright, "The Nature of Group Cohesion," p. 91.
7. Alvin Zander, *Motives and Goals in Groups* (New York: Academic Press, Inc. 1971), p. 174.
8. Cartwright, "The Nature of Group Cohesion," p. 104.
9. J.W. Thibaut and H.H. Kelley, *The Social Psychology of Groups* (New York: Wiley, 1959), p. 98.
10. Rensis Likert, *New Patterns in Management* (New York: McGraw-Hill Book Co., 1961), p. 103.
11. _____, *The Human Organization* (New York: McGraw-Hill Book Co., 1967), pp. 4-10.
12. Harish C. Jain, "Internal Communications and Supervisory Effectiveness in Two Urban Hospitals" (Madison, Wisc.: Ph.D. diss., University of Wisconsin, 1970), pp. 90-91.
13. Ibid., p. 93.
14. Ibid., p. 94.
15. Ibid., pp. 95-101.

SUGGESTED READINGS

Exline, R. "Group Climate as a Factor in the Relevance and Accuracy of Social Perception." *Journal of Abnormal and Social Psychology* 55: 382-388.

Guion, R.M. "A Note on Organizational Climate." *Organizational Behavior and Human Performance* 9: 120-125.

James, L.R., and Jones, Allen P. "Organizational Climate: A Review of Theory and Research." *Psychological Bulletin* 81, no. 12: 1096-1112.

Johannesson, R.E. "Some Problems in the Measurement of Organizational Climate." *Organizational Behavior and Human Performance* 10: 118-144.

Kehoe, P.T., and Reddin, R. *Organizational Health Survey*. Fredericton, N.B., Canada: Organizational Test Limited.

LaFollette, W.R., and Sims, H.P. "Is Satisfaction Redundant With Climate?" *Organizational Behavior and Human Performance* 13: 252-278.

Lawler, E.E.; Hall, Douglas T.; and Oldham, Greg R. "Organizational Climate: Relationship to Organizational Structure, Process, and Performance." *Organizational Behavior and Human Performance* 11: 139-155.

Lee, C. "Organizational Climate: A Laboratory Approach," Masters' thesis, Department of Communication, Ohio State University, 1975.

Litwin, G., and Stringer, R. *Motivation and Organizational Climate*. Boston: Harvard University Press, 1967.

Lott, A., and Lott B. "Group Cohesiveness, Communication Level, and Conformity." *Journal of Abnormal and Social Psychology* 62: 408-412.

Pepitone, A. and Reichling, G. "Group Cohesiveness and the Expression of Hostility." *Human Relations* 8: 327-343.

Perrow, C. "Hospitals: Technology, Structure, and Goals." In *Handbook of Organizations*, edited by J. March, Chapter 8. Chicago: Rand McNally, 1965.

Pritchard, R.D., and Karasick, B. "The Effect of Organizational Climate on Managerial Job Attitudes and Job Satisfaction." *Organizational Behavior and Human Performance* 9: 126-146.

Raven, B., and Rietsema, J. "The Effect of Varied Clarity of Group Goal and Group Path Upon the Individual and His Relationship to His Group." *Human Relations* 10: 29-44.

Van Zelst, R. "Sociometrically Selected Work Teams Increase Production." *Personnel Psychology* 5: 175-186.

Willerman, B., and Swanson, L. "Group Prestige in Voluntary Organization." *Human Relations* 6: 57-77.

CLIMATE REVIEW PUZZLE

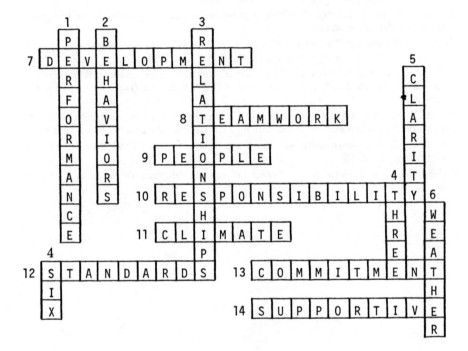

DOWN

1) A major climate dimension.
2) Determines organizational climate.
3) Affected by organizational climate.
4) Number of performance dimensions.
5) A performance dimension.
6) Similar to but different from organizational climate.

ACROSS

7) A major climate dimension.
8) A development dimension.
9) Who creates organizational climate?
10) A development dimension.
11) A collective organizational view.
12) A performance dimension.
13) Another performance dimension.
14) Highly motivated individuals tend to work in _____ organizational climates.

Chapter 3

Improved Supervision through Deliberative Listening

CHAPTER OBJECTIVES

The purpose of this chapter is to enable you to CHANGE your communicative behavior in a *positive* direction. After studying the material you should be able to:

Communicate more effectively through the development of good listening habits.

Heighten your ability to understand other people through better listening.

Assess your listening ability.

Name and apply appropriate listening responses.

Gain the belief that listening can be improved.

Eradicate poor listening habits.

INTRODUCTION

One of our first experiences with education was the first day we were sent off to school. One of the exciting times in this period in our lives was when we were told to bring an object to class and tell the class about it. This may have been our first experience with public speaking. The following years were devoted to endless classes in reading, writing, and arithmetic; but probably the most important of all skills was overlooked—the art of listening.

Bill Conboy has said that listening is a skill. Listening proficiency can be improved with practice. It is not a static condition like the shape of your nose or feet. Research in both business and education has demonstrated that most individuals can improve in listening performance.[1]

Warren Ganong of the Methods Engineering Council compared trainees who had knowledge of listening skills to those who had no knowledge. Those with listening-skill knowledge achieved marks 12 to 15 percent higher than those with no knowledge.[2]

Many employees feel that they are paid to do a job and the job requires doing. However, they overlook the importance that listening plays in doing a job well. Listening can mean greater efficiency. Listening stems from the need to gather necessary data. Listening helps in settling grievances. Listening makes people feel special.

Many companies are recognizing the value of effective listening and have added courses in listening to their training programs. A few of these companies are American Telephone and Telegraph, General Motors Corporation, The Dow Chemical Company, Minnesota Mining and Manufacturing, International Business Machines, and Western Electric.

DELIBERATIVE LISTENING

Charles Kelly has defined deliberative listening as a unitary skill, the ability to hear information, to analyze it, to recall it at a later time, and to draw conclusions from it. In deliberative listening, one strives to understand the message for the purpose of using the information contained in the message.[3]

Listening Requires Time and Energy

Although, in the form of "self-talk," we spend a great deal of time listening to ourselves, at times we don't even do that well. About 70 percent of our working day is spent in verbal communication. Research shows that average working adults divide their communication time roughly along these lines:[4]

Listening	45%
Talking	30%
Reading	16%
Writing	9%

These statistics indicate that almost one-half of our communication time is spent in listening. A failure to listen not only affects the relationships between hospital supervisors and employees, but also the quality of health care given the patient. Before reading further, think carefully and write down your own personal definition of the word "communication." How you define that word will tell you something about you as a listener.

At the seventh annual Hospital Topics Supervisor Management Conference, held in 1979 in Chicago, supervisors were asked to write down their personal definition of the word "communication." Some of those in attendance defined communication as the process of sending messages. This definition emphasized the sending aspect of communication and overlooked the importance of the need for a receiver (listener). Just because a message was sent does not mean it was received or listened to. To have good communication, someone must take the time and effort to listen to and understand what has been said. The hospital supervisor who defines communication simply as a process of sending messages might be inclined to say,

- "I'm the supervisor, and I don't have time for a lot of silly questions," or
- "I told the employee what I meant. Why can't he understand that?"

Other supervisors at the conference defined communication as the process of sending *and* receiving messages. They understood that in order to have good communication there must be deliberative listening that evolves into interaction, exchange of information, and understanding. These respondents focused on the receiving or listening aspects of the communicative act.

When something is extremely important, there is a need for a communication check. The supervisor must find out if the message was listened to. Was it received the way it was intended to be received? Was there a transfer of common meaning? The hospital supervisor who is concerned with communication in this manner might say,

- "To answer the employee's question, I have to listen to what is being asked;"

- "Good communication is when I understand what the employee has said;" or

- "Communication is effective when I listen to what my employees have to say and when they listen to what I have to say."

Your personal definition of communication, which you have written down, expresses your attitude toward the listening aspect of communication. If you defined communication with emphasis on the receiving end as well as the sending end, you recognized the importance of listening.

Upon closer examination, we discover that it is the listening side of the communicative act that enables us to gather the necessary data to solve problems, to settle a grievance, to become more efficient, to build a supportive climate, or to make a person feel special.

Feedback

During examinations, the doctor and nurse do not tell patients how they should feel. The patient sends messages, and the doctor and nurse receive feedback through listening. By this we are not referring to a situation in which someone has you for dinner and two weeks later you have them over for a "feedback." The term *feedback* refers rather to the *certified mail* of communication. It enables one to make sure that the message that was transmitted was received the way it was intended to be received.

Thus, it can be said that feedback is characterized in these ways:

Facilitates communication.

Enables the sender to make sure that the transmitted message was received the way it was intended to be received.

Empathy is required.

Descriptive rather than evaluative.

Both verbal and nonverbal.

Avoid misunderstandings.

Can help persons to change their behaviors.

Keeps communication channels open.

Feedback must always be, even in confrontations, the positive side of the negative, adding to understanding rather than subtracting from the receiver's self-esteem. It provides the opportunity for increased understanding of the messages that are sent and received. However, the effectiveness of feedback is dependent upon the sender of the message. If truthful messages are not being sent, the feedback that is returned will be inaccurate, which may prove to be detrimental to the individual or to the group. Feedback should always be directed toward some behavior that the receiver can do something about. Frustration is only increased when a person is reminded of some shortcoming over which that person has no control.

Listening Responses

One of the deceptive features of listening behavior stems from our comparative lack of feedback with respect to how we are doing. A listening response is a very brief comment or action made to another person to convey the idea that the recipient is interested, attentive, and wants the person to continue. The response is made quietly and briefly, so as not to interfere with the speaker's train of thought. It is usually made when the speaker pauses. There are five types of listening responses:

Nod: Nodding the head slightly and waiting.
Pause: Looking at the speaker expectantly.
Casual remark: "I see." "Uh-huh." "Is that right?"

Query: Asking genuine questions.
Paraphrasing: Repeating back to the speaker your understanding
                  of what has been said.

It has been suggested that each communicative act can involve at least six interpretations:

Message-Sender

1. What another person means to say.
2. What the other person hears himself or herself saying.
3. What another person actually says.

Receiver-Listener

4. What you hear the other person actually saying.
5. What you hear the other person saying.
6. What the other person says means to you.

As you listen, how do you attempt to deal with this? Here is a suggestion to use the next time you are listening to an employee in a discussion, debate, or argument. Before you reply to the employee's comments, repeat what the employee has said. In turn, before the employee replies to your comment, he or she should repeat what you have said. This process will be both an eye and an ear opener.

Finally, can improved listening skills improve not only your own ability to listen but also the ability of others to listen? In this area, common sense tells us that no one can force others to do something they don't want to do. The most that you can hope for is that your behavior will act as a model for others to emulate. A particular kind of behavior normally brings about a like behavior. If I like you, there will be at least a chance that you will like me. If I don't like you, there is little chance that you will like me. It is the same with listening. If you listen to someone, there is at least the possibility that that person will also listen to you.

Health care supervisors and employees who can improve their listening ability can make significant contributions to the health care team. Only by listening to one another can we share our dreams, hopes, and fears and exchange ideas. This sharing is what makes a team—a group working together toward a common goal: improved patient care.

HOW DO YOU RATE AS A LISTENER?

Take the following test and see how you rate as a listener. Place an "X" in the appropriate blank. When speaking interpersonally with a patient, nursing supervisor, doctor, coworker, or employee, do you:

Usually   *Sometimes*   *Seldom*

			(1) Prepare yourself physically by standing or sitting, facing the speaker, and making sure you can hear?
___	___	___
___	___	___	(2) Watch the speaker for the verbal as well as the nonverbal messages?
___	___	___	(3) Decide from the speaker's appearance and delivery whether or not what he or she has to say is worthwhile?
___	___	___	(4) Listen primarily for ideas and underlying feelings?
___	___	___	(5) Determine your own bias, if any, and try to allow for it?
___	___	___	(6) Keep your mind on what the speaker is saying?
___	___	___	(7) Interrupt immediately if you hear a statement you feel is wrong?
___	___	___	(8) Try to see the situation from the other person's point of view?
___	___	___	(9) Try to have the last word?
___	___	___	(10) Make a conscientious effort to evaluate the logic and credibility of what you hear?

SCORING

This check list, though by no means complete, should help you measure your listening ability. Score yourself as follows: Questions 1, 2, 4, 5, 6, 8, and 10—ten points for *usually,* five points for *sometimes,* and zero points for *seldom.* Questions 3, 7, and 9—zero points for *usually,* five points for *sometimes,* and ten points for *seldom.*

If you scored below 70, your listening skills can be improved because you have developed some undesirable listening habits; 70 to 85, you listen well but can still improve; 90 or above, you are an excellent listener.

People tend to do things well when they hold positive views or "labels" about their ability to do it. You can't do it until you think you can. There is a human tendency to live up or down to labels. If you think you are a good listener, you probably are, and, because of this positive label, you make a conscientious effort to listen, to live up to your label. If you say you are a poor listener, you have turned off your listening mechanism. You must think you can do it before you attempt to do it. If you fail to try because of your fear of failure, you may never discover your hidden potential.

At a recent workshop, a nurse approached one of the authors after taking a tape-recorded listening test and remarked, "If I hadn't done well on that test, I would have been very disappointed, because I consider myself to be an excellent listener." In other words, she scored as an excellent listener, and her positive attitude toward listening played a key role in her listening effectiveness.

CHECKLIST OF GUIDELINES TO IMPROVE LISTENING SKILLS

The following ten guidelines, in conjunction with the test you just took, should provide a more comprehensive basis to improve your listening skills:

1. You should prepare yourself physically by standing or facing the speaker. Making sure you can hear physically is essential for good listening. You thereby tell the sender that you are ready to listen and are able to hear the verbal messages and also see the nonverbal messages the speaker is sending. This face-to-face attention also shows that you are interested in what is being said. People tend to avoid and look away from people and things in which they are not interested. Attention and interest are synonymous. You pay attention to the things you are interested in, and you are interested in the things you pay attention to.

2. You should learn to watch for the speaker's nonverbal as well as verbal messages. Everyone sends two messages. One message is sent verbally, and the other is sent nonverbally through inflection in the voice or through facial expression, bodily action, or gestures. Sixty-eight percent of all messages are sent nonverbally. The nonverbal message conveys the speaker's attitude, sincerity, and genuineness. To miss the nonverbal message is to miss half of what is being said.

3. You should not decide from the speaker's appearance or delivery that what he or she has to say is worthwhile. When you start to focus on the speaker's delivery or appearance, you become distracted from the purpose of communication: receiving the speaker's ideas. You should be more interested in what people have to say than how they say it or what they look like.

4. You should listen for ideas and underlying feelings. Again, the purpose of good communication is to be able to reflect upon and exchange ideas. For example, if I were to meet you on the street and give you a dollar and you gave me a dollar, and you then went your way and I went mine, neither of us would be better off because of the exchange. But if I gave you an idea and you gave me an idea, then both of us would be better off as a result of the exchange.

5. You should try to determine your own biases, if any, and allow for them. Communication gets blamed for many things. Whenever something doesn't go right, you might say you have a communication breakdown. But many times you don't have a communication breakdown at all. In fact, you might have very good communication; you both know what has been said, and there is a common understanding. But you don't like what you have heard. If the health care supervisor or employee could learn to recognize such differences, better relationships would be formed. You will not always agree with everyone. The trauma in such situations develops when you discover you are no longer talking about the issues, but about each other.

6. You should attempt to keep your mind on what the speaker is saying. Don't allow yourself to become distracted. Too many times, people fake attention and, like the little dog in the back of the car window, just keep nodding their heads up and down without hearing a word of what is being said.

7. You should not interrupt immediately if you hear a statement that you feel is wrong. Indeed, if you listen closely, you may be persuaded that the statement is right. Sometimes you may fail to listen just because of this fear of something different, of the possibility that you may have to forsake some sacred position you have held for years.

8. You should try to see the situation from the other person's point of view. This doesn't mean that you always have to agree. However, there is no way that you can change other people's perceptions until you can see how they have formulated those perceptions.

9. You should not try to have the last word. Listen to what is being said, and then think about it. This reflection may take some time, but you need time to think before you communicate. Sometimes, in order to solve a problem, you have to walk away from the problem for a while and think about it from different points of view, and about the advantages and disadvantages of possible solutions.

10. You should make a conscientious effort to evaluate the logic and credibility of what you hear. Our minds function at some 500 words a minute, but we normally speak at 125 words a minute. In other words, we can think four times faster than we can speak. Rather than letting our minds become bored, we can take advantage of this time differential between thinking and speaking. We can attempt to anticipate the speaker's next point, attempt to identify and evaluate supporting material, and mentally summarize what the speaker has said: What has thus far been said that I can use?

Remember, listening makes the people you are listening to feel special; sometimes it enables them to solve their own problems. Perhaps they are in the process of hearing themselves think aloud on a subject for the first time. At such times, they might just want others to listen. If you refrain from injecting yourself into the conversation, you might be able to help them resolve their own internal conflicts.

As a professional or supervisor, you are paid to listen. Yet studies at the University of Minnesota, confirmed by studies at Florida and Michigan State Universities, showed that people forget one-third to one-half of what they hear within eight hours.[5]

The art of listening is a skill, however, and it can be improved. You listen best when you develop a positive attitude toward listening. The first step is to become aware of the fact that listening is not a passive activity. Also, there is little correlation between intelligence and listening. You must "want" to remember.

One technique that supervisors can use to improve their listening ability is to pretend that they will be quizzed later in the day about what they have heard. The health care professionals and supervisors who improve their listening ability can make significant contributions to their health care teams.

DELIBERATIVE LISTENING REVIEW PUZZLE

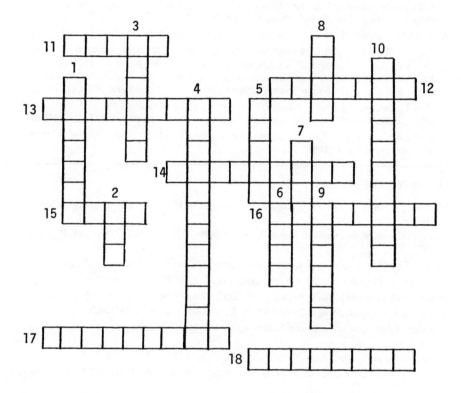

DOWN

1) Due to speed differential.
2) One type of listening response.
3) Can be reduced through good listening.
4) Can improve listening.
5) Can determine behavior.
6) A reason we may not listen.
7) Number of types of listening responses.
8) Approximate amount of time spent listening.
9) Good listening is an _____.
10) In deliberative listening we strive to _____ messages.

ACROSS

11) A type of listening response.
12) How we spend 30 percent of our communication time.
13) Sixty-eight percent of all messages.
14) Is needed to solve problems.
15) Functions at 500 words per minute.
16) The certified mail of listening.
17) Fifty percent of the communicative act.
18) A synonym for attention.

(Answers on page 55.)

NOTES

1. Bill Conboy, *Working Together: Communication in a Healthy Organization* (Columbus, Ohio: Charles E. Merrill Publishing Co., 1976), p. 73.
2. Ralph G. Nichols, "Listening Is a Ten Part Skill," *Nation's Business*, July 1957, p. 56.
3. Charles M. Kelly, "Actual Listening Behavior of Industrial Supervisors as Related to Listening Ability, General Mental Ability, Selected Personality Factors and Supervisory Effectiveness," *Small Group Communication: A Reader*, ed. Robert S. Cathcart and Larry A. Samovar (Dubuque, Iowa: William C. Brown Co., Publishers, 1970), pp. 251-259.
4. Paul T. Rankin, "Listening Ability," *Proceedings of the Ohio State Educational Conference, Ninth Annual Session* (Columbus, Ohio: Ohio State University, 1929), pp. 172-183.
5. J.H. Kramar and T.R. Lewis, "Comparison of Visual and Nonvisual Listening," *Journal of Communication* 1 (1951): 16.

SUGGESTED READINGS

Barbara, Dominick A. *The Art of Listening*. Springfield, Ill.: Charles C. Thomas, Publisher, 1966.

_____. *How to Make People Listen to You*. Springfield, Ill.: Charles C. Thomas, Publisher, 1971.

Barker, Larry L. *Listening Behavior*. Englewood Cliffs, N.J.: Prentice Hall, Inc., 1971.

Byrne, Donn P. *Listening*. New York: Longman, Inc., 1975.

Duker, Sam. *Listening Bibliography*. New York: Scarecrow Press, Inc., 1964.

_____. *Listening Readings*. Metuchen, N.J.: Scarecrow Press, Inc., 1964.

Erickson, Allen G. "Can Listening Efficiency Be Improved?" *Journal of Communication* 4, no. 4: 53.

Kerman, Joseph. *Listen*. New York: Worth Publishing Co., 1976.

Mills, Ernest P. *Listening: Key to Communication*. New York: Petrocelli Charter, Inc., 1974.

Nichols, Ralph G. "Listening Is a Ten Part Skill." *Nation's Business*, July 1957, pp. 56-60.

_____, and Stevens, Leonard A. *Are You Listening?* New York: McGraw-Hill Book Co., 1957.

_____, and Stevens, Leonard A. "If Only Someone Would Listen." *Journal of Communication* 6, no 1: 8.

_____, and Stevens, Leonard A. "Listening to People." *Harvard Business Review*, September-October 1957, pp. 85-92.

Rogers, Carl R., and Farson, Richard E. *Active Listening*. Chicago: Industrial Relations Center, University of Chicago, 1955.

Strong, Linda. "Do You Know How to Listen?" *Management Review* 44: 530-535.

Toussaint, Isabella H. "A Classified Summary of Listening, 1950-1959." *Journal of Communication* 10: 125-134.

Whyte, W.H., Jr. *Is Anybody Listening?* New York: Simon and Schuster, 1952.

Zelko, Harold P. *How To Be A Good Listener*. New York: Employee Relations, 1958.

_____. "An Outline of the Role of Listening in the Communication Process." *Journal of Communication* 4: 71.

DELIBERATIVE LISTENING REVIEW PUZZLE

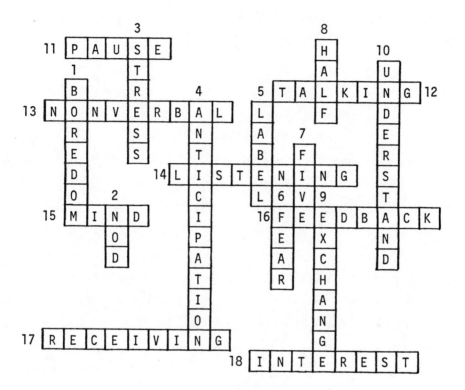

DOWN

1) Due to speed differential.
2) One type of listening response.
3) Can be reduced through good listening.
4) Can improve listening.
5) Can determine behavior.
6) A reason we may not listen.
7) Number of types of listening responses.
8) Approximate amount of time spent listening.
9) Good listening is an _____.
10) In deliberative listening we strive to _____ messages.

ACROSS

11) A type of listening response.
12) How we spend 30 percent of our communication time.
13) Sixty-eight percent of all messages.
14) Is needed to solve problems.
15) Functions at 500 words per minute.
16) The certified mail of listening.
17) Fifty percent of the communicative act.
18) A synonym for attention.

Chapter 4

Improved Supervision through Active Listening

CHAPTER OBJECTIVES

The purpose of this chapter is to enable you to CHANGE your communicative behavior in a *positive* direction. After studying the material you should be able to:

Comprehend the importance of active listening.

Have an understanding of the prerequisites for active listening.

Actively listen for feelings.

Name the attending and responding functions of active listening.

Guide others toward more effective listening.

Eliminate the dysfunctional styles of responding.

The authors express their appreciation to Dr. Rebecca Leonard for the material contained in this chapter on pages 59-66 from her paper, "Active Listening: Skilled Interpersonal Communication," published June 1979, Raleigh, North Carolina, © Rebecca Leonard, 1979.

INTRODUCTION

A Marine Corps general was visiting an installation and asked to see the bugler privately. "Can you play fire call?" he inquired. "Yes, sir," replied the marine. "Then meet me tomorrow at 5 A.M. in front of the post headquarters and don't mention this to anyone," said the general.

The post commander was so eager to know what was going on that he pressured the bugler into telling him about his conversation with the general. That night the post's fire station was a beehive of activity as equipment was washed and polished. Even the door hinges were oiled. The next morning the marine bugler reported to the general.

"Sound church call," the general ordered.

"But, sir, you asked me if I knew fire call."

"Yes, son, I know, but now please play church call!"

As the first notes pierced the early morning stillness, the doors of the fire station flew open and out roared the trucks with bells clanging and sirens screaming.

Good listening habits are not the easiest of skills to develop, and that may be why many of us do it so poorly. Too many times we develop mental sets or preconceived ideas as to what is being said. We hear the other person, but we are not listening. Often we miss the *real* message. We fail to recognize the feelings that are not articulated by words. We are not actively involved in what is being said.

To be a good listener requires intense concentration. Research has shown that people involved in active listening show degrees of tension as they try empathically to understand what has been said.

Active listening requires the development of skills, just as deliberative listening does. It requires above all that you not be passive. Richard Weaver has stated: "It is an active, not a passive process. We cannot just make sure that our ears are alert or open and let the rest come naturally. Because active listening involves both emotional and intellectual inputs, it does not just happen. We have to make it happen. It takes energy and commitment."[1]

An interesting analogy between breathing habits and listening habits has been postulated by Bill Conboy:

> Doctors and biologists agree that breathing is one life process which human beings tend to handle poorly. It has been estimated that most of us could add 10 to 15 years to

our life span if we practiced better breathing habits from an early age. Yet breathing is one thing we do throughout our lives. Listening habits, like breathing habits, improve only with systematic and evaluated practice. Real listening requires an expenditure of energy in obtaining and retaining the spoken discourse of others. Tests in the physiological psychology laboratory have shown that active listening demands as much energy, makes a person just as tired, as comparable efforts in speaking, reading, or writing.[2]

Active and deliberative listening requires energy plus a desire to understand. Yet the two types of listening are as different as they are similar. Charles Kelly explains that the desired result of the two types is similar—the accurate understanding of verbal communication. But this understanding is achieved in different ways:

The deliberative listener "first" has the desire to critically analyze what the speaker has said, and "secondarily" tries to understand the speaker. . . . The active listener has the desire to understand the speaker "first" and, as a result, tries to take appropriate action. This does not mean to suggest that the active listeners are uncritical or always in agreement with what is communicated, but rather that their primary interest is to become fully and accurately aware of what is going on.[3]

THE IMPORTANCE OF ACTIVE LISTENING

Active listening plays an important role in supervisor-employee relationships, but it is also important in relationships between neighbors, roommates, friends, parents, children, teachers, and students. Unfortunately, active listening is not highly valued in our society. It is brushed aside by many of us who were taught to listen only in the deliberative style. It should be remembered, however, that we do not listen only with our ears. We also listen with our eyes and our sense of touch; we listen by becoming aware of the feelings and emotions that arise within us because of our contact with others. We listen with our mind, our heart, and our imagination.

Good active listening requires that we listen for all possible meanings—those behind the words as well as the obvious meanings. Richard Weaver suggests:

To listen effectively we have to pay attention to facial expressions and eye contact, gestures and body movements, posture and dress, as well as the quality of the other person's voice, vocabulary, rhythm, rate, tone, and volume. . . . listening with our third ear helps us to understand the whole message.[4]

This suggestion is especially applicable to the supervisor-employee relationship. To be effective, the supervisor must actively listen for feedback. The supervisor must be able to listen to all meanings, of what has been said and in some cases of what has been left unsaid. The supervisor should remember that even silence can be communication. When employees refuse to communicate with their supervisors or coworkers, they are sending all kinds of messages. We cannot not communicate.

PREREQUISITES FOR ACTIVE LISTENING

Before the skills of active listening can be learned, certain preconditions must be met. Carl Rogers and Richard Farson believe that the good listener must meet four prerequisites in order to experience a mutually beneficial interaction:

1. The listener must *want* to listen.
2. The listener must be willing to *suspend judgment;* that means accepting the other person. This does not mean that the listener must approve of all the behaviors or attitudes of the other person; it means, however, that such approval or disapproval must be suspended throughout the interaction. If the other person is to deal with the problem responsibly, the good listener cannot make judgments or offer advice.
3. The listener must allow and *encourage* a statement of feelings by the other person. In order to solve problems successfully, such feelings must be acknowledged, accepted, and felt.
4. The listener must be *aware* of personal feelings during the interaction and must be prepared to integrate them into the interaction when appropriate.[5]

Rogers notes that "the major barrier to mutual interpersonal communication is our very natural tendency to judge, to evaluate, to approve or disapprove, the statement of the other person."[6]

He goes on to say that "real communication occurs, when this evaluated tendency is avoided, when we listen with understanding. What does this mean? It means to see the expressed idea or attitude from the other person's point of view, to sense how it feels to him, to achieve his frame of reference in regard to the thing he is talking about."[7]

SKILLS IN ACTIVE LISTENING

Once the prerequisites of active listening are met, the listener is psychologically ready to listen. This psychological preparation is not yet enough, however, to achieve fully the promise of good listening. The achievement of empathy is important, but the listener must also communicate that empathy through "attending" and "responding." Gerard Egan has noted that "if I am to let you know that I understand you, I must first pay attention to you and listen to what you have to say about yourself."[8]

Here are some of the attending (nonverbal) and responding (verbal) behaviors by which an active listener expresses empathy.

*Attending (nonverbal)**	*Responding (verbal)**
• Facing the other person squarely	• Evaluative responses
• Adopting an open posture	• Interpretive responses
• Leaning toward the other person	• Supportive responses
• Maintaining good eye contact	• Probing responses
• Being relatively relaxed	• Understanding responses
• Reflecting attention through facial expressions	
• Attending with vocal cues	

Attending Responses

The nonverbal cues that indicate that the listener is *attending* are primarily physical: facing the other person squarely, adopting an open posture, leaning toward the other person, maintaining good

---

Source: Adapted from Gerard Egan, *You and Me: The Skills of Communicating and Relating to Others,* Monterey, Calif.: Brooks-Cole Publishing Co., 1977, pp. 114-115; and David W. Johnson, *Reaching Out: Interpersonal Effectiveness and Self Actualization,* Englewood Cliffs, N.J., Prentice-Hall, Inc., p. 125.

eye contact, maintaining a relatively relaxed musculature, and reflecting attention through appropriate facial expressions.

Egan believes that your body can either emphasize the message you are trying to communicate with words or it can erase the message you are sending with words and even substitute an opposite message.[9]

Albert Mehrabian noted the following division of the communicative process. He discovered that, of the total message, 7 percent is verbal, 38 percent is vocal, and 55 percent is facial.[10] Mehrabian's findings emphasize the importance of the 93 percent of the message that is nonverbal. He also notes that such nonverbal attending behaviors are indications of *caring*, manifested in immediacy or liking.[11]

Becoming aware of the nonverbal is important to supervisors as they attempt to listen. First, they can become sensitive to the value of their own verbal cues in communicating to the employee sending the message that they are listening. Supervisors can say through their attention, "We are here, we are interested in you, we want to listen." Attending thus confirms for the sender that listening is occurring. Second, supervisors as listeners can become sensitive to the *total* message of the sender through attention to the latter's nonverbal as well as verbal cues. Supervisors' recognition of both the verbal and nonverbal parts of messages will aid them in developing understanding and empathy.

Responding Responses

Though paying attention is important, it does not always lead to accurate, empathic understanding between sender and listener. It is also important to let other people know how you interpret their messages.

John Stewart and Gary D'Angelo call this process "perception checking." They state: "When you are perception checking, you verbalize your interpretation or inferences about what was said or left unsaid, and you ask the other person to verify or correct your interpretation."[12]

Perception checking allows us to at least attempt to develop common meaning. A common poster in most speech departments states:

I Know That You Believe You Understand What You
Think I Said, but, I Am Not Sure You Realize
That What You Heard Is Not What I Meant.

Phrasing of Responses

Stewart and D'Angelo suggest two categories of responses: paraphrasing and parasupporting.[13] There are four rules of paraphrasing:

1. Say in your own words what you heard the other person saying.
2. Try to include some of what you perceive the other person to be feeling.
3. Don't just "word swap." That is, do not merely repeat what the sender has said. Repeating does little to let the sender know that the listener understands. Nor does it really encourage the sender to elaborate.
4. Give the other person a chance to verify your paraphrase.

Even attentive and active listeners are not always accurate in their interpretations. The purpose of perception checking is to determine whether or not the sender's message has been accurately interpreted and understood. If the listener has misinterpreted the sender, the good listener will admit it. Few senders will be fooled by a dishonest listener; but most will in fact appreciate an honest mistake, and the listener's trustworthiness will be enhanced.

The second dimension of perception checking suggested by Stewart and D'Angelo is parasupporting. Here, listeners will not only paraphrase what the senders have said but will also carry their own ideas further by providing examples or other data that tend to illustrate, clarify, or support the senders' feelings.[14]

DYSFUNCTIONAL STYLES OF RESPONDING

In the development of an appropriate response style, the listener might have the tendency to respond in dysfunctional ways. Egan offers eight examples:

1. *The cliché.* When someone discloses a personal problem, a response with a cliché such as, "Oh, I know how you feel," can be less functional than no response at all. Egan believes that clichés put distance between people.

2. *The question.* A question can be helpful in probing, that is, in gaining information concerning the sender's problems. But a question can also be perceived as interrogation and place the other person on the defensive. With few exceptions, a question can be rephrased into a declarative statement. The purpose of gaining information is thus still served, but the possibility of defensiveness is avoided.

3. *Inaccuracy.* If your understanding of other people is unaccurate, those people may feel "blocked," that is, they may lose trust in your ability to understand and, as a result, stop the interaction. Perception checking can help the listener avoid inaccuracies.

4. *Feigning understanding.* It isn't always easy to understand what a sender is trying to communicate, even if the listener "attends" well. But if the listener merely pretends to understand, the sender will sense this, and this will create a barrier. Egan says, "If you are confused admit your confusion. . . . Such statements are signs of respect, of the fact that you think it is important to stay with the other."[15]

5. *Parroting.* Mere repetition of what the other person says does little to establish empathy.

6. *Jumping in too quickly or letting the other person ramble.* The good listener will let the other person pace the interaction, unless that person begins to ramble. Listeners should feel free to interrupt if they have something important to say, but generally the senders should be in charge.

7. *Discrepancy in language, tone, or manner.* The use of idiosyncratic jargon or behavior by the listener is inappropriate. As far as possible, the listener should follow the cues from the sender so the sender does not feel invaded.

8. *Longwindedness.* The listener's responses should be as succinct as possible. Comments should be to the point, but not too long. Remember, the sender is in control of the interaction.[16]

Other common mistakes in listening noted by Egan are indicated by the following types of responses:

- responses that imply condescension or manipulation
- unsolicited advice giving
- responses that indicate rejection or disrespect
- premature confrontation

- patronizing or placating responses
- responses that ignore what the person said
- use of inappropriate warmth or sympathy
- judgmental remarks
- defensive responses[17]

SUMMARY

The following advice is offered to improve your "deliberative" and "active" listening ability:

- Most of us talk too much. At times we should use judicious silence. Silence is a great way to motivate other people to speak up, to let us know what's on their minds.

- Most of us frame questions to get the answers we want to hear. We should frame our questions so that we leave the way open for whatever type of answer the other person wants to give. We should allow the other person time to finish the answer.

- Most of us set up communication in counterproductive atmospheres. If possible, we should pick a time and place that provide maximum comfort and minimum distraction. If the communication is an emotion-laden issue, we should pick a place of privacy and protect the dignity of all parties.

- Many of us let emotional filters get in the way of understanding. Be honest about your biases. When you feel strongly about a subject, be particularly careful. At such times there is a chance that you will misinterpret, misunderstand, and miscommunicate. The next time your emotions boil over, make a mental note regarding the time and place and people involved. You might be able to track down the source of your feelings and the trigger that sets you off.

- Most of us listen only for facts. We fail to see the topic from the other person's point of view. Listen for feelings. Pay as much attention to the way you or someone else says something as to what is said. Pay attention to *all* meanings. Then check out your perceptions with these phrases: "I conclude that you approve (or disapprove) of . . . ," or "Am I right in concluding that what you are saying is . . . ?"

It cannot be overemphasized that listening only for facts can severely delimit one's ability to understand what is *really* being said. Ultimate awareness can only take place if we allow our intuition to come into focus. Sometimes it is best to *lose your mind and come to your senses.*

An anonymous poet has written:

> *A wise old bird sat on an oak,*
> *The more he saw the less he spoke,*
> *The less he spoke the more he heard,*
> *Lord, make me like that wise old bird.*

ACTIVE LISTENING REVIEW PUZZLE

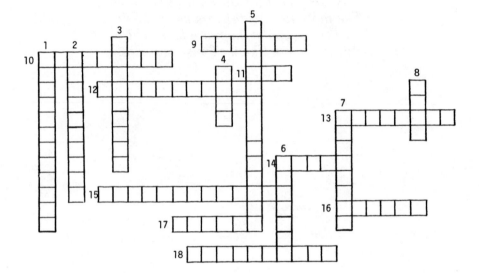

DOWN

1) A dimension of perception checking.
2) Displaying verbal listening behaviors.
3) Displaying nonverbal listening behaviors.
4) Number of paraphrasing rules.
5) A dimension of perception checking.
6) Shown by people involved in active listening.
7) The certified mail of listening.
8) The listener must _____ to listen.

ACROSS

9) Requirement for active listening.
10) A dysfunctional response.
11) We should listen for _____ meanings.
12) These should be checked.
13) Important in solving problems.
14) We should listen with our _____ ear.
15) Should be avoided.
16) A dysfunctional response.
17) What attending behaviors indicate.
18) A poor listening attitude.

(Answers are on page 71.)

NOTES

1. Richard Weaver, *Understanding Interpersonal Communication* (Glenview, Ill.: Scott, Foresman and Co., 1978), p. 100.
2. Bill Conboy, *Working Together: Communication in a Healthy Organization* (Columbus, Ohio: Charles E. Merrill Publishing Co., 1976), pp. 73-74.
3. Charles M. Kelly, "Actual Listening Behavior of Industrial Supervisors as Related to Listening Ability, General Mental Ability, Selected Personality Factors and Supervisory Effectiveness," *Small Group Communication: A Reader*, ed. Robert S. Cathcart and Larry A. Samovar (Dubuque, Iowa: William C. Brown Co., Publishers, 1970), pp. 252-253.
4. Weaver, *Understanding Interpersonal Communication*, p. 99.
5. Carl R. Rogers and Richard E. Farson, "Problems in Active Listening," *Communication Probes*, ed. B.D. Peterson, G.M. Goldhaber, and R.W. Pace (Chicago: SRA, 1974), pp. 30-34.
6. Carl R. Rogers, *On Becoming a Person* (Boston: Houghton Mifflin Co., 1961), p. 330.
7. Ibid., pp. 331-332.
8. Gerard Egan, *You and Me: The Skills of Communicating and Relating to Others* (Monterey, Calif.: Brooks-Cole Publishing Co., 1977), p. 109.
9. Ibid., p. 113.
10. Albert Mehrabian, *Silent Messages* (Belmont, Calif.: Wadsworth Publishing Co., 1971), p. 43.
11. Ibid., pp. 1-23.
12. John Stewart and Gary D'Angelo, *Together: Communicating Interpersonally* (Reading, Mass.: Addison-Wesley, 1975), p. 192.
13. Ibid., p. 195.
14. Ibid., p. 193.
15. Gerard Egan, *Interpersonal Living* (Monterey, Calif.: Brooks-Cole Publishing Co., 1976), pp. 124-129.
16. Ibid.
17. Ibid., p. 131.

SUGGESTED READINGS

Barbara, Dominick A. "On Listening: The Role of the Ear in Psychic Life." *Today's Speech* 5, no. 1: 12-15.

Bird, D.E. "Have You Tried Listening?" *Journal of the American Dietetic Association* 30: 225-230.

Brown, C.T. "Studies in Listening Comprehension." *Speech Monographs* 26: 288-294.

Kelly, C.M. "Emphatic Listening." In *Small Group Communication: A Reader*, edited by R.S. Cathcart and L.A. Samovar. Dubuque, Iowa: William C. Brown Company, Publishers, 1970.

Nichols, Ralph G. "Factors in Listening Comprehension." *Speech Monographs* 15: 154.

Reik, Theodor. *Listening with the Third Ear*. New York: Grove Press, 1948.

Rogers, Carl R., and Farson, Richard E. *Problems in Active Listening.* Chicago, Ill.: Industrial Relations Center, University of Chicago, 1974.

––––––, *On Becoming a Person.* Boston: Houghton Mifflin Company, 1961.

Weaver, Carl H. *Human Listening: Processes and Behavior.* New York: Bobbs-Merrill Company, Inc., 1972.

ACTIVE LISTENING REVIEW PUZZLE

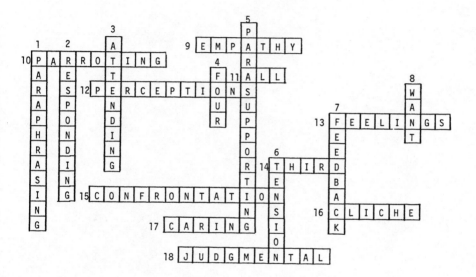

DOWN

1) A dimension of perception checking.
2) Displaying verbal listening behaviors.
3) Displaying nonverbal listening behaviors.
4) Number of paraphrasing rules.
5) A dimension of perception checking.
6) Shown by people involved in active listening.
7) The certified mail of listening.
8) The listener must _____ to listen.

ACROSS

9) Requirement for active listening.
10) A dysfunctional response.
11) We should listen for _____ meanings.
12) These should be checked.
13) Important in solving problems.
14) We should listen with our _____ ear.
15) Should be avoided.
16) A dysfunctional response.
17) What attending behaviors indicate.
18) A poor listening attitude.

Chapter 5

The Dynamics of
Supervisory Leadership

CHAPTER OBJECTIVES

The purpose of this chapter is to enable you to CHANGE your communicative behavior in a *positive* direction. After studying the material you should be able to:

Compare the differences between the interactional and trait approaches of leadership.

Have an understanding of the *task* and *maintenance* functions of leadership.

Assess your knowledge of leadership.

Notice leadership potential in others.

Generate a *new* style of personal leadership.

Evaluate your own leadership ability.

INTRODUCTION

Little can be accomplished without some predetermined plan of action. In fact, by definition, to accomplish means to meet a goal. To reach goals requires leadership. Thus, to meet early twentieth century goals, most organizations were directed by autocratic or paternalistic leaders. Workers were willing to listen and respond to the boss and the expert. Now, in the latter half of the century, workers are more apt to question authority. This questioning attitude on the part of workers is commonly referred to as the psychology of job entitlement.

In the early part of the twentieth century, the problem of leadership did not seem as severe as it is today. In politics, business, and education, certain people were designated as *the* experts; and voters, employees, and students tended to think of the world as being divided into leaders and followers. In short, our society was much less complex than it is today.

In the last ten years, however, Los Angeles has grown by 2.5 million. In July 1964, the population of the United States was about 192 million. The U.S. Census Bureau estimates that the population in 1980 was approximately 222 million. Today, more than half of all Americans were born after World War II and are under 35 years of age.

Forty years ago, only one out of every eight Americans had gone to high school. Today, four out of five attend high school. Forty years ago, less than 4 percent of the population attended college. Now the figure is around 40 percent. These changes have stimulated new approaches to the study of leadership.

There have been more than 1800 studies of leadership, but there is still little agreement on how to describe, identify, or evaluate it. Leadership effectiveness has many different dimensions; effective leaders must meet the interpersonal needs of the group members they lead.

Early research on leader effectiveness was centered on the leader. Gradually, however, the concept of group dynamics emerged from the social sciences with a focus primarily on members of the group rather than solely on the leader.

The new approach stemmed primarily from Kurt Lewin and his associates in the late 1930s and early 1940s. The group dynamics movement stressed the larger human element rather than merely the thinking element in group behavior. This larger emphasis provided researchers with new insights into the interactions between leader and follower.

TASK AND INDIVIDUAL BEHAVIOR

Andrew Halpin notes that there are two main components of leadership—task and individual behavior—that appear to play significant roles in the interaction between leaders and followers.[1]

Other writers refer to the needs of group members in defining task and individual behavior. William Sattler and N. Edd Miller believe that task-oriented leaders deal with problem-solving functions; they ask to have goals identified, ask for information, give information, evaluate information, resolve differences, and call for plans of action. The task-oriented leader is mainly interested in getting the job done, regardless of personal feelings.[2]

On the other hand, leaders oriented toward individuals show a willingness to reveal signs of friendliness, warmth, respect, and mutual trust. Through this type of behavior, leaders can attempt to eliminate their followers' feelings of anxiety, strain, tension, embarrassment and discomfort.[3]

R.F. Bales refers to these two leadership dimensions as reciprocal or opposite pairs:

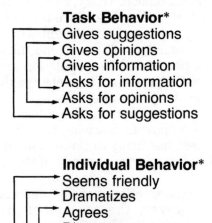

Task Behavior*
Gives suggestions
Gives opinions
Gives information
Asks for information
Asks for opinions
Asks for suggestions

Individual Behavior*
Seems friendly
Dramatizes
Agrees
Disagrees
Shows tension
Seems unfriendly

**Source:* Adapted from R.F. Bales, *Personality and Interpersonal Behavior,* New York: Holt, Rhinehart, and Winston, 1970, p. 92.

It should be kept in mind that the dimensions of task and individual behavior are not mutually exclusive categories. The components of task-oriented behavior and individual-oriented behavior tend to cross-stimulate one another.

A hospital supervisor can exhibit only four possible combinations of behavior:

1. High task and high individual behavior (HTHI)
2. High task and low individual behavior (HTLI)
3. High individual and low task behavior (HILT)
4. Low task and low individual behavior (LTLI)

In Chapter 2 we discussed the importance of a positive group climate. Here, it must be emphasized that the leader plays a key role in the development of such a climate. Staff motivation and morale will be determined, to a large extent, by the type of task and individual behaviors the leader exhibits within the work group. Research studies indicate that employees derive a higher level of job satisfaction when their leaders exhibit high task and high individual behavior.

THE LEADER AND THE GROUP

Richard Heslin and Dexter Dunphy prepared detailed abstracts of 450 small group studies and then analyzed those studies that dealt with group satisfaction. Their findings were that member satisfaction is high when (1) either a leader emerges who is effective in both the task and individual functions of the group, or two complementary leaders emerge with one handling the task functions and the other handling the individual functions; and (2) the designated leader or leaders are perceived by the group members to be competent.[4]

As noted earlier, the two supervisory leadership behaviors are not mutually exclusive. The supervisor should remember that the dual role of leadership sometimes requires movement away from democratic, group-centered leadership toward autocratic leadership. On the other hand, the supervisory leader's belief in the democratic process, in the ability of the members of the group to solve their own problems, tends to pull the supervisory leader back to group-centered, democratic leadership. When the need for both approaches is recognized, the leader will be suited to the group and the situation.

PRODUCTIVITY AND JOB SATISFACTION

The Institute of Social Research at the University of Michigan has conducted numerous studies in an attempt to find out what makes an organization tick and, more specifically, how the principles and practices of leadership bear directly on the productivity and job satisfaction of various groups. These studies conclude that:

- It is not necessarily true that a favorable attitude among employees toward the company will result in increased productivity.

- When comparing people under general supervision (where the goal to be accomplished is clear and the employees are given leeway in accomplishing it) with persons under close supervision (where the supervisor is constantly in attendance and permits little leeway for the subordinates), those groups under close supervision tend to be associated with low productivity while those under more general supervision show higher productivity.

- Supervisors of high productivity groups more often report that they are kept informed of developments than do supervisors of low productivity groups.

- When work groups with the lowest and highest morale were asked to describe what their supervisors did, workers in low morale groups mentioned just as often as workers in high morale groups that their supervisors performed such production-centered tasks as "enforces the rules," "arranges work and makes work assignments," and "supplies men with materials and tools." But the high morale groups mentioned much more frequently than the low morale groups such employee-centered functions as "recommends promotions and pay increases," "informs men on what is happening in the company," "keeps men posted on how they are doing," and "hears complaints and grievances."

- There is a marked relationship between worker morale and how strongly employees feel that their boss is interested in discussing work problems with the work group.

- The high production groups show greater group loyalty and greater group pride than do the low production groups.

- When supervisors were asked, "How does your section compare with other sections in the way men help one another on the job?" the answers showed a marked relationship to productivity. Supervisors of high production groups reported more often than supervisors of low production groups that their workers helped one another in getting the work done.[5]

You may recall from Chapter 2 that the group climate is the collective view of the people within an organization regarding the nature of the environment in which they work. The climate of a group plays a key role with respect to the group's level of productivity and member satisfaction. The climate is dependent upon both the leadership and the workers of the organization. It may initially appear that the leader plays a minor role in the establishment of group climate. This is not the case; the leader, by focusing attention on factors of group climate, can change that climate very rapidly.

The establishment of a positive group climate that stimulates employee motivation and heightens staff morale will be determined by how the leader's task and individual behaviors are combined in the group.

Hanan Selvin has studied the differences between what he called *persuasive climate* and *arbitrary climate*. He points to the need to establish a climate of psychological safety and refers to the dual roles of leadership and how each of these factors influences the other. He found that persuasive climates reduced tension and tended to satisfy personal needs more than arbitrary climates. He also found that a personal nonthreatening climate improved task efficiency.[6]

Carl Rogers poses the hypothesis that group members identify with their leader and in the process internalize some of their leader's characteristics of leadership. This might mean that members of a group will begin to behave toward other group members in much the same way their leader behaves toward them. They would become more friendly and warm toward others in the group, more empathic in their relations with others, if their leader's behavior was also oriented toward this end.[7]

THE LEADERSHIP SELECTION PROCESS

Most social psychologists and experts in communication agree on certain basic characteristics of leadership. Before we proceed to establish criteria for leadership selection, see how closely you agree with the experts by taking this brief test. Decide whether each statement is more true or more false. The answers and test rationale will be given later in the chapter.

True   *False*

_____	_____	1. Leaders are born, not made.
_____	_____	2. Leadership should be a reward for loyalty or length of service.
_____	_____	3. Only extroverts can be effective leaders.
_____	_____	4. You can tell leaders by their neat appearance.
_____	_____	5. The more automatic and habitual the thinking and action of leaders, the more democratic their leadership will become.
_____	_____	6. Effective leaders often forget about a problem for a while in order to solve it.
_____	_____	7. A leader with a deep interest in people will normally be more effective than a leader who is only interested in getting the job done.
_____	_____	8. Leaders are best suited to select future leaders.
_____	_____	9. In most cases, how people behaved in the past will determine their future behavior.
_____	_____	10. Leadership effectiveness is dependent upon the situation.

The Trait Approach

One of the earliest approaches used to select leaders was called the trait approach. It attempted to list characteristics that "good" leaders had in common. These traits might be enthusiasm, friendliness, direction, integrity, skill, intelligence, courage, and so on. For many years, it was believed that good leaders could be identified by observing their characteristics, that certain traits set leaders apart from other people who were not destined to be leaders. An examination of the studies on leadership, however, reveals the major weakness of the trait approach: seldom do the suggested lists of traits agree on the essential elements of leadership.

R.M. Stogdill surveyed over 100 studies of leadership. He discovered that less than five percent of the traits reported as effective leadership characteristics were common in four or more of the studies surveyed. He also found evidence that suggested that leaders cannot be too different from their followers and that followers must be able to identify with their leaders.[8]

The Interactional Approach

The early studies on leadership depended entirely upon specific leadership traits and tended to disregard the importance of interaction between leader and follower. However, the staff of the Ohio State Leadership Studies discovered as a result of its investigations that it is more important to speak of the *leader behavior* of people rather than their leadership capacity or ability. This allows one to speak about what people do when they are leading. When leadership is thought about in this way, attention is focused on the interaction of people and the roles they play in a group situation. This approach thus appears to be more meaningful than the trait approach in selecting leaders.

In the interactional approach, the leadership behaviors or acts are identified, and the group interactions can be described quite reliably. In contrast, the trait approach provides little assurance that persons having certain traits—such as personality, skill, ability, or intelligence—could be depended upon to lead in all situations. The trait approach examines only the *static* characteristics of people; it does not describe the *dynamics* of leadership as a process.[9]

Thus, research has more recently centered on observing behavioral patterns within work groups. From opinions, observations, tests, and intensive research into the actual process of supervision, the following job behaviors of successful supervisory leaders have emerged. Successful managers

- manage work instead of people
- plan and organize effectively
- set goals realistically
- derive decisions by group consensus, but accept responsibility for them
- delegate frequently and effectively
- rely on others for help in solving problems
- communicate effectively

- are a stimulus to action
- coordinate effectively
- cooperate with others
- show consistent and dependable behavior
- win gracefully
- express hostility tactfully[10]

The interactional approach can best be summarized in the following points:

- Leadership is a product of the interaction that takes place among individuals in a group; it is not a product of the status or position of these individuals.
- Activity by an individual that tends to clarify thinking, create better understanding, or otherwise cause group action is called leader behavior or leader activity.
- The effectiveness of leader behavior is measured in terms of mutuality of goals, productivity, and the maintenance of group solidarity.

Of course it is rarely possible to be all things to all people. Every supervisory leader knows that in most work groups a small percentage of employees cause most of the problems.

Lawrence Steinmetz has quoted former General Motors president Edward Cole as stating:

> . . . a research study found that a relatively few employees—28%—filed 100% of the grievances and accounted for 37% of the occupational hospital visits, 38% of the insurance claims, 40% of the sick leaves, 52% of the garnishments, and 38% of the absenteeism experienced at a certain factory. Thus are there not only a comparatively small proportion of people who are absentee oriented, but these same people tend to also be the ones who create a significant number of all the other problems generated within the organization.[11]

KEY POINTS FOR THE SUPERVISORY LEADER

Every supervisor has a responsibility to exhibit leadership behavior when the situation warrants it. The following key points will make you more effective as a supervisory leader:

- Do you attempt to see the other person's point of view? This doesn't mean, Do you always agree with the other person?

- You have more status than you think you have. This status derives from employees' perceptions of their immediate supervisors. To the average employee in your department, you are the boss.

- Can you disagree with an employee without being disagreeable?

- You are often the person in the middle, but still you can arrive at a productive and efficient relationship with the people you supervise.

- Do you listen to and not just hear your employees? There is a real difference between listening and hearing; listening suggests that you are at least trying to understand how the other person feels about things.

- Consultation can be of enormous assistance to you in getting people to do their jobs.

- Are you responsible? When an employee asks you to do something, and you can, do you follow through?

- Two-way communication is essential for the modern supervisor.

- Can you be trusted? When you say something to your employees, will they believe it?

- Successful supervision is not constant supervision. Know your people and give to each employee what is needed in the way of instruction, information, and evaluation.

- Can your employees identify with you in some way? Are you one of them working toward a common goal?

- Remember there are two pay systems: the normal pay system based on competitive wages and fair differentials, and the other pay system which includes appreciation, communication, and opportunity for fulfillment.

- Do you give your employees the opportunity to express their ideas?

- Many of your employees desire more challenging work. Productive and efficient employees should not be *hoarded* by the supervisor. Provide opportunities for advancement and more challenging work, even if this means a transfer out of your department.

- Are you enthusiastic? Can you transfer that enthusiasm to your employees?

- The supervisor who moves into higher positions in the institution is more often than not a people-centered supervisor, one who has obtained results through appreciating and understanding employees' needs.

- Do you encourage employees in doing a good job?

- Participation is essential to the success of a work team. The supervisor achieves participation by encouraging subordinates to make suggestions. Such encouragement is enhanced by a nonjudgmental attitude toward suggestions and a willingness to explore the feasibility of all suggestions.

- If you are going to succeed in the modern work arena—with its complex challenges produced by changes in our society, higher expectations from employees, and a more educated work group—you must move from a supervisory style anchored in authority and obedience to one based on involvement, participation, and commitment.

- Most important, are you more interested in the welfare of your employees and the organization than in personal recognition?

Leadership Style Questionnaire

This is not a test with right or wrong answers. It is a questionnaire designed to describe some of your attitudes about leadership. It contains ten statements about situations. After each statement, there are three possible behaviors or actions indicated that you might take if placed in a position of leadership. Place a number 3 beside the position you would *most likely* take, a number 2 beside the position you would *next likely* take, and a number 1 beside the position you would *least likely* take.

For each question you should have three answers: a 3 for your preferred behavior or action, a 2 for your second choice, and a 1 for your least likely choice.

---

1. *In leading a meeting it is important to:*

   - keep the focus on the agenda at hand .... (1) _____
   - focus on each individual's feelings and help people express their emotional reactions to the issue ..... (2) _____
   - focus on the differing perceptions people have and how they deal with each other .... (3) _____

2. *A primary objective of a leader is:*

   - to maintain an organizational climate in which learning and accomplishment can take place .... (4) _____
   - to maintain the efficient operation of the organization (5) _____
   - to help members of the organization find themselves and be more aware of who they are .... (6) _____

3. *When strong disagreement occurs between a leader and a group member about work to be done, the leader should:*

   - listen to the person and try to discover how that person might have misunderstood the task .... (7) _____
   - try to get other people to express their views in order to involve them in the issues .... (8) _____

- support the group member for raising the question or
  disagreement .... (9) _____

4. *In evaluating a group member's performance, the leader should:*

   - involve the entire group in setting goals and in evaluating one another's performance .... (10) _____

   - try to make an objective assessment of each person's accomplishments and effectiveness .... (11) _____

   - allow individual members to be involved in determining their own goals and performance standards .... (12) _____

5. *When two group members get into an argument, it is best to:*

   - help them deal with their feelings as a means of resolving the argument .... (13) _____

   - encourage other members to respond to the argument and to try to help resolve it .... (14) _____

   - allow some time for expression of both sides, but keep in focus the relevant subject matter and the task at hand .... (15) _____

6. *The best way to motivate group members who are not performing up to the best of their ability is to:*

   - point out to them the importance of the job to be done and their role in it .... (16) _____

   - try to get to know them better so you can understand why they are not realizing their potential .... (17) _____

   - show them how their lack of motivation is affecting other people .... (18) _____

7. *The most important element in judging group members' performance is:*

   - their technical skill and ability .... (19) _____

- how they get along with their peers and how they help others learn and get the work done .... (20) ____
- their success in meeting the goals they set for themselves .... (21) ____

8. *In dealing with minority group issues, a leader should:*

- deal with such issues as they threaten to disturb the atmosphere of the work group .... (22) ____
- be sure that all group members understand the history of racial and ethnic minorities in the community and country .... (23) ____
- help group members to achieve an understanding of their own attitudes toward people of other races and cultures .... (24) ____

9. *A leader's goal should be to:*

- make sure that all group members have a solid foundation of knowledge and skills that will help them become productive and effective people .... (25) ____
- help people to learn to work effectively in groups, to use the resources of the group, and to understand their relationships with one another as people .... (26) ____
- help group members become responsible for their own education and effectiveness .... (27) ____

10. *The trouble with leadership responsibilities is that:*

- they make it very difficult to cover adequately all the details that must be attended to .... (28) ____
- they keep a leader from really getting to know group members as individuals .... (29) ____
- they make it difficult for the leader to keep in touch with the climate and pulse of the group .... (30) ____

SCORING

Note that, in scoring the questionnaire, the scoring columns are not in the usual sequential order.

SCORING COLUMNS

INSTRUCTIONS

	TASK	INDIVIDUAL	CLIMATE

1. Transfer your answers from the Leadership Style Questionnaire to the scoring columns at right, placing a 1, 2, or 3 beside each question number.

	TASK	INDIVIDUAL	CLIMATE
	(1)____	(2)____	(3)____
	(5)____	(6)____	(4)____
	(7)____	(9)____	(8)____
	(11)____	(12)____	(10)____
	(15)____	(13)____	(14)____
	(16)____	(17)____	(18)____
	(19)____	(21)____	(20)____
	(23)____	(24)____	(22)____
	(25)____	(27)____	(26)____
	(28)____	(29)____	(30)____
	TOTAL____	TOTAL____	TOTAL____

2. Add up your totals for each column. The three totals combined should equal 60.
3. Mark your score for each dimension on the bar graph below. Blacken in the bar from the left to your score on each dimension.
4. The completed bars represent your leadership profile at this moment in time.

|←——low——→|←——high——→|

			TASK			
			INDIVIDUAL			
			CLIMATE			
0	5	10	15	20	25	30

HOW TO INTERPRET YOUR LEADERSHIP PROFILE

1. Three bars of similar length (within variations of two or three points) indicate that you try to balance your concerns for task, feelings, and climate.
2. The longest bar tends to symbolize your characteristic leadership style in most situations. This style is probably functional for you most of the time, but it may be overused.
3. The shortest bar indicates an area you may tend to overlook. You might improve the situation by placing more emphasis on the leadership style represented by that bar.
4. You will improve your leadership the fastest by attending to issues symbolized by the shorter bars.

SUPERVISORS COMPOSITE LEADERSHIP STYLE PROFILE

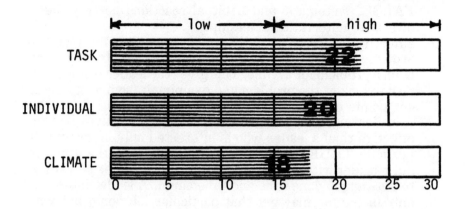

You may now wish to compare your leadership style profile with the composite profile obtained at the seventh annual *Hospital Topics* Conference held in Chicago in 1979.

Earlier in this chapter you were asked to take a test on your knowledge of leadership. The answers to the ten questions and their rationale are presented below:

1. Leaders are born not made. FALSE. Research indicates that environmental factors and proper training play a significant role in the development of leadership abilities.
2. Leadership should be a reward for loyalty or length of service. FALSE. Only the most sincere, energetic, and capable individuals who have a desire to serve should be appointed to positions of leadership. Loyalty is important, but leadership requires more than just loyalty.
3. Only extroverts can be effective leaders. FALSE. To be a leader, one must have visibility. However, many reserved and quiet people exhibit tremendous leadership ability when given the opportunity to express themselves.
4. You can tell leaders by their neat appearances. FALSE. We should be more interested in what leaders do when they are leading. Their ideas, their attitudes, their ability to motivate others are more important than the first impressions they make.

5. The more automatic and habitual the thinking and action of leaders, the more democratic their leadership will become. FALSE. Automatic and habitual reactions portray highly directive, autocratic leadership.
6. Effective leaders often forget about a problem for a while in order to solve it. TRUE. Sometimes it is best to walk away from a problem for a while. This gives the leader the opportunity to look at the problem and examine it from many different points of view.
7. A leader with a deep interest in people will normally be more effective than a leader who is interested only in getting the job done. TRUE. Leadership does depend upon the situation, but a leader with a deep interest in people will be better able to get the job done time and time again. A leader interested only in the job may get that particular job done, but what about the next job?
8. Leaders are best suited to select future leaders. FALSE. Research has shown that leaders should be selected by how well they work and interact with the people they are to lead. Appointed leaders may work well with the person who appointed them, but how do they work with the people they are to lead? A leader must have followers, for without followers there is no need for a leader.
9. In most cases, how people behaved in the past will determine their future behavior. TRUE. Remember, the statement applies to *most cases* and does not mean to suggest that a person cannot ever change. On the other hand, if a person has been a hard worker and reliable and conscientious over a long period of time, the chances that that person will stay that way are pretty good.
10. Leadership effectiveness is dependent upon the situation. TRUE. A leader cannot always respond to everyone in the same way. The behavior of leaders will be determined to a large extent by the attitudes and training of their followers.

If you scored nine or ten of the statements correctly, you are going in the right direction and have an excellent awareness of the meaning of leadership. If you scored seven or eight correctly, you are at times uncertain about the way to go, and you have some misconceptions about leadership that may limit your ability to lead effectively. If you scored less than seven correctly, you need to work on your leadership awareness and capabilities.

LEADERSHIP REVIEW PUZZLE

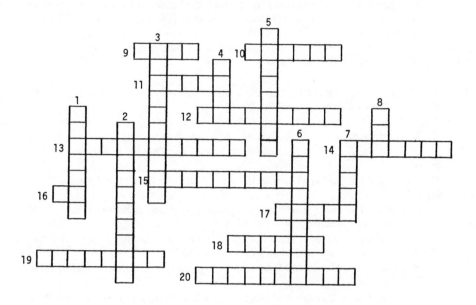

DOWN

1) A collective group view.
2) A necessary element in order to achieve a group goal.
3) Highly directive leadership.
4) Initials of behavior for ideal leadership.
5) Needed to implement change in existing policies.
6) Leaders must have these.
7) They accurately perceive interpersonal needs.
8) The number of major leadership components.

ACROSS

9) Behavior that emphasizes getting the job done.
10) Those whom a leader leads.
11) An approach used to pick leaders.
12) A variable that leadership is dependent upon.
13) What a leader should encourage in a group.
14) A way to conceive of the role of leadership.
15) Behavior that emphasizes human conditions.
16) Initials of behavior indicating little job interest.
17) Should be determined by the leader and the group together.
18) Effective leaders do this often.
19) Group energy.
20) An "individual" kind of behavior.

(Answers are on page 94.)

NOTES

1. Andrew Halpin, "Evaluation Through the Study of the Leader's Behavior," *Perspectives on the Group Process*, ed. C. Kemp (Boston: Houghton-Mifflin Professional Publishers, 1964), pp. 264-265.

2. William Sattler and N. Edd Miller, *Discussion and Conference* (Englewood Cliffs, N.J.: Prentice Hall Inc., 1968), pp. 213-214.

3. Ibid.

4. Richard Heslin and Dexter Dunphy, "Three Dimensions of Member Satisfaction in Small Groups," *Human Relations* 17 (1964): 99-112.

5. Rensis Likert, *Motivation: The Core of Management, Personnel Series No. 155* (New York: American Management Association, 1953), pp. 3-20.

6. Hanan C. Selvin, *The Effects of Leadership* (Glencoe, Ill.: Free Press of Glencoe, 1960), p. 45.

7. Carl Rogers, *Client Centered Therapy* (Houghton-Mifflin Professional Publishers, 1951), pp. 348-349.

8. R.M. Stogdill, "Personal Factors Associated with Leadership: A Survey of the Literature," *Journal of Psychology* 25 (1948): 64.

9. William Alexander, *Leadership for Improving Instruction* (Washington, D.C.: Association for Supervision and Curriculum Development, 1960), p. 109.

10. J.P. Campbell et al., *Managerial Behavior, Performance and Effectiveness* (New York: McGraw-Hill Book Co., 1970), p. 8.

11. Lawrence Steinmetz, *Managing the Marginal and Unsatisfactory Performer* (Reading, Mass.: Addison-Wesley, 1969), pp. 10-11.

SUGGESTED READINGS

Bass, Bernard. *Leadership Psychology and Organizational Behavior.* New York: Harper & Row, 1960.

Bennett, Addison. "New Thinking Required for Development of Management Effectiveness." *Hospitals* 50: 67-70.

Bittel, Lester R. *What Every Supervisor Should Know.* 2nd ed. New York: McGraw Company, 1968.

Blake, Robert R., and Mouton, Jane Srygley. *The Grid for Supervisory Effectiveness.* Austin, Texas: Scientific Methods, Inc., 1975.

Fiedler, Fred E., and Chemers, Martin. *Leadership and Effective Management.* Glenview, Ill.: Scott, Foresman and Co., 1974.

Gordon, Thomas. *Leadership Effectiveness Training.* New York: Wyden Books, 1977.

Kuriloff, Arthur H. "An Experiment in Management: Putting Theory Y to the Test." *Personnel* 40: 8-17.

Liberman, Robert P.; King, Larry W.; DeRisi, William J.; and McCann, Michael. *Personal Effectiveness: Guiding People to Assert Themselves and Improve Their Social Skills.* Champaign, Ill.: Research Press, 1975.

McMurray, Robert M. "Are You the Kind of Boss People Want to Work For?" *Business Management* 28: 59-60.

Myers, M. Scott. *Every Employee a Manager: More Meaningful Work Through Job Enrichment.* New York: McGraw-Hill Book Co., 1970.

Nealy, S.M., and Blood, M.R. "Leadership Performance of Nursing Supervisors at Two Organizational Levels." *Journal of Applied Psychology* 52: 120-129.

—————, and Owen, T.M. "A Multitrait-Multimethod Analysis of Predictors and Criteria of Nursing Performance." *Organizational Behavior and Human Performance* 5: 348-365.

Peter, Lawrence. *The Peter Principle.* New York: Morrow, 1969.

—————. *The Peter Prescription.* New York: Morrow, 1972.

Pfiffer, John M. *The Supervision of Personnel: Human Relations and the Management of Men.* 2nd ed. Englewood Cliffs, N.J.: Prentice-Hall, Inc., 1958.

Phelps, Stanley, and Austin, Nancy. *The Assertive Woman.* San Luis Obispo, Calif.: Impact Press, 1975.

Preston, M., and Heinz, R. "Effects of Participatory Versus Supervisory Leadership on Group Judgment." *Journal of Abnormal and Social Psychology* 44: 345-355.

Stogdill, R.M. "Personal Factors Associated with Leadership: A Survey of the Literature." *Journal of Psychology* 25: 35-71.

Townsend, Robert. *Up the Organization.* New York: Alfred A. Knopf, Inc., 1970.

LEADERSHIP REVIEW PUZZLE

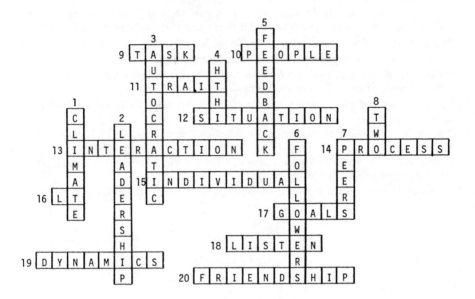

DOWN

1) A collective group view.
2) A necessary element in order to achieve a group goal.
3) Highly directive leadership.
4) Initials of behavior for ideal leadership.
5) Needed to implement change in existing policies.
6) Leaders must have these.
7) They accurately perceive inter-personal needs.
8) The number of major leadership components.

ACROSS

9) Behavior that emphasizes getting the job done.
10) Those whom a leader leads.
11) An approach used to pick leaders.
12) A variable that leadership is dependent upon.
13) What a leader should encourage in a group.
14) A way to conceive of the role of leadership.
15) Behavior that emphasizes human conditions.
16) Initials of behavior indicating little job interest.
17) Should be determined by the leader and the group together.
18) Effective leaders do this often.
19) Group energy.
20) An "individual" kind of behavior.

Chapter 6

The Supervisor's Use of Nonverbal Communication

CHAPTER OBJECTIVES

The purpose of this chapter is to enable you to CHANGE your communicative behavior in a *positive* direction. After studying the material you should be able to:

Comprehend the fact that you are constantly sending nonverbal messages.

Have an understanding of the nonverbal variables that affect relationships.

Assess the nonverbal messages of your patients, coworkers, and employees.

Note that nonverbal behavior is culturally derived.

Gain an ability to recognize and be able to respond to nonverbal feedback.

Examine nonverbal meaning.

INTRODUCTION

As a supervisor, how often have you heard a coworker or employee say, "Seeing is believing. Did you see the way he acted when I said . . . ?" Or, "I can tell by the look on her face," Or "I knew he would act that way!" All of these statements reflect a belief that the nonverbal message expresses the truth more than the verbal message. Sometimes we miss the nonverbal messages that are sent to us, indicating "I don't understand;" "Leave me alone;" "Help me, I'm depressed;" or "I think I understand, but tell me more."

Gail and Michelle Myers point to the important role that nonverbal communication plays in our daily interactions with others:

> You communicate nonverbally through the inflection of your voice, your tone, your pitch; you use gestures, facial expressions to communicate a whole range of meanings to the people you interact with. You also communicate nonverbally through your clothes and the objects with which you surround yourself. Touching is a very significant part of your communication repertoire, and the rules you follow about whom to touch, where to touch, how frequently to touch, and in which situations to touch are heavily based on cultural factors. Time and space are important features of the communication system you use with others. Proxemics, or the study of distance, can be useful in helping you understand the relational dimension of your interpersonal communication. Nonverbal communication is often used to express feelings and emotions. If the messages you receive through the verbal system do not seem to fit other messages you receive through the nonverbal system, you usually rely on the nonverbal dimension of communication to interpret what was really meant. Nonverbal messages help you to verify the intentions of other speakers and also reinforce their other messages.[1]

NONVERBAL FEEDBACK

Nonverbal feedback provides supervisors with a tool to discriminate more accurately between what is being said verbally and what is *really* being said nonverbally. The insight gained from such feedback enables supervisors to anticipate problems and to help employees to the extent that the supervisors are able to recognize and respond to nonverbal feedback.

Everyone sends two messages at the same time. People send one message verbally and the other message nonverbally, through facial expression, eye contact, bodily action, and use of space. When the nonverbal message and the verbal message are congruent, we tend to have clear, meaningful communication. However, when the nonverbal message appears to contradict the verbal message, we tend to have unclear and faulty communication.

Ray Birdwhistell noted in the Paul Swain Lecture Series at North Carolina State University that

> Body language and spoken language are dependent on each other. Spoken language by itself will not give us the full meaning of what a person is saying. Body language alone will not give us total meaning. If we listen to only the words the person is saying, we may get as much distortion as if we only listen to the body language. However, 55 percent of the social meaning in a conversation is transmitted nonverbally, and in its proper context even silence is communication.[2]

Employees may choose to stop talking, but they do not cease to communicate. Have you ever tried to talk to employees, but they refused to talk to you, or at best said very little, and you desperately needed more information? You may not have realized it, but those employees were sending you all kinds of nonverbal messages. To quote Sigmund Freud: "No mortal can keep a secret. If his lips are silent he chatters with his finger tips; betrayal oozes out of him at every pore."[3]

Helmut Mossback notes that too many times silences are overlooked, but when viewed in their proper context those silences can take on significant meaning.

> An American professor at a Japanese university with an excellent command of the Japanese language attended a meeting where he fully participated in the lengthy discussions, using Japanese throughout. On leaving the meeting, he remarked to a Japanese colleague that, in his opinion, the meeting had finally arrived at a particular conclusion. Had not Professor X spoken in favor? His Japanese col-

league agreed. And other professors, too? (going down the list one by one). Again, his Japanese colleague agreed, but finally remarked, "All this may be so, but you are still mistaken. The meeting arrived at the opposite conclusion: You have correctly understood all the words spoken, but you didn't understand the silences between them.[4]

THE IMPACT OF NONVERBAL MESSAGES

Nonverbal behaviors normally have a high degree of credibility in the mind of the beholder. Most hospital employee recruiters tend to agree. "I make up my mind fast in less than five minutes," stated one hospital employee recruiter. "Sometimes I take a second look, but seldom change my mind." The same sentiment was expressed at a recent workshop of the North Carolina Directors of Hospital Personnel Services. One director said, "I look for nonverbal cues to support what is being said. My first impression is based on appearance, facial expression, eye contact, and gestures. A sloppy applicant is at a disadvantage, especially at hospitals that don't have dress codes. I believe that clothing is an extension of self and the nonverbal behavior of the applicants truly expresses their personality and attitude."

E.C. Webster found that interviewers formed an initial impression of an applicant within the first four or five minutes of the interview and then tended to search for additional information that supported and substantiated their initial impressions.[5]

Mehrabian found in situations he examined that only 7 percent of the total impact of the communication was verbal. Another 38 percent was based on how the words were said (paralanguage); and the remaining 55 percent was based on facial expression, gestures, and bodily action.[6]

FORMS OF NONVERBAL COMMUNICATION

Facial Expressions

More than 100 years ago, Charles Darwin wrote *The Expression of Emotions in Man and Animals*, the product of a century-old pursuit and one of the first works on facial expression.[7] Darwin theorized that facial expressions are instinctive and not learned behavior. However, today most anthropologists believe that facial expressions are a result of natural reactions in the muscles and nerves of the face and of cultural conditioning that governs the expression of emotion.

In the American culture, facial expressions play an important role in the social communications between people. Facial expressions can convey true feelings and be useful communicative tools. Unfortunately, however, the general rule regarding facial expressions in America seems at times to parallel that of the ancient Greek Stoics, in that we are taught from childhood to avoid excessive expressive behavior, facial or otherwise. We are taught to show neutrality when we are angry, especially in a public place. If we are unhappy, we are urged to show only the slightest sense of sadness in our demeanor. In our culture, and in many others, false facial expressions can be masks behind which we hide.

However, even with these limitations, the face is one of the most reliable of all nonverbal indicators. Mark L. Knapp, noting the importance of the face as an indicator, states that "the face is rich in communicative potential. It is the primary site for communication of emotional states; it reflects interpersonal attitudes; it provides nonverbal feedback on the comments of others; and some say it is the primary source of information next to human speech."[8]

There are six basic facial expressions: disgust, surprise, happiness, anger, sadness, and fear. Several of these expressions can be exhibited at the same time. An employee can simultaneously exhibit surprise and disgust or surprise and happiness.

The problem of interpretation is compounded when the verbal message seems to be in conflict with the facial expression. Most nonverbal theorists agree that, if the meaning of the facial expression is clear and the verbal context in which it occurs is not, the face will be the most reliable source.

P. Ekman, W. V. Friesen, and P. Ellsworth conducted an indepth analysis of all the important studies of facial expression and concluded: "Contrary to the impressions conveyed in previous reviews of the literature that the evidence in the field is confusing and contradictory, our reanalysis showed consistent evidence of accurate judgment of emotion from facial behavior."[9]

A. Mehrabian and M. Weiner found that, when exposed to an inconsistent message, facial expression has the greatest impact, vocal expression has the second greatest, and verbal expression has the lowest impact.[10]

Eye Contact

A look is more than just seeing. Meaning is constantly being conveyed in numerous visual ways—through the stern look of a boss, the loving look of a patient's relative, or the cooperative look of coworkers. Eye contact is a highly personalized form of nonverbal communication.

As early as 1921, G. Simmel reported:

> The union and interaction of individuals is based upon mutual glances. This mutual glance between persons, in distinction from the simple sight or observation of the other, signifies a unique union between them. By the glance which reveals the other, one discloses himself. . . . The eye cannot take unless at the same time it gives.[11]

Michael Argyle surmises that we spend between 30 to 60 percent of the time exchanging mutual glances with others. He believes there are several implicit rules about interacting visually:

- A looker might invite interaction by staring at another person who is on the other side of the room. The target's studied return of the gaze is generally interpreted as acceptance of the invitation, while averting the eyes is a rejection of the looker's request.

- There is more mutual eye contact between friends than others, and a looker's frank gaze is widely interpreted as positive regard.

- Persons who seek eye contact while speaking are regarded not only as exceptionally well-disposed by their target, but also as more believable and earnest.

- If the usual short, intermittent gazes during conversation are replaced by gazes of longer duration, the target interprets this as meaning that the task is less important than the personal relations between the two persons.[12]

Eye contact tells us how we are doing and the kind of relationship we have with another person. We tend to look at things we like and to look away from things we dislike. Michael Argyle and Janet Dean discovered that a speaker's eye contact occurs at the end of phrases and sentences but does not occur during long statements. When two people like one another, they establish eye contact more often and for longer duration than when there is dislike or tension in the relationship.[13]

Paralanguage

It has often been said by college debaters that it's not what you say that counts, but how you say it. The tone of the voice conveys different types of meaning. Our telephone conversations, for example, rely heavily on paralanguage. The inflection in the voice, the pauses, and the rate of speech can convey anger, happiness, boredom, interest, love, hate, frustration, or uncertainty. Telephone conversations do not allow us the luxury of seeing gestures, facial expressions, or bodily actions.

During interpersonal communication with employees, we rely heavily on paralanguage to determine the genuineness of the message. Myers and Myers cite the following examples of verbal statements and what they might really mean, depending on the paralanguage that is being used:

- Verbal: "I'll be happy to do it."
  Paralanguage: "I'll do it, but it will be the last time."

- Verbal: "You always make me do what you want."
  Paralanguage: "All right, you win."

- Verbal: "Don't worry, I'll take care of it."
  Paralanguage: "You're so dumb I better take care of it."[14]

It should be emphasized that paralanguage (vocal inflection) is the second most important of those indicators of nonverbal meaning that ultimately determine the impact of the message being received.

Bodily Action

To a large extent, a person's social identity and self-image are created by bodily actions. Abne Eisenberg and Ralph Smith state that "each person's psychic well being depends upon manipulating the image which he presents to others. That is, the individual's definition of himself is shaped and sustained by the reaction of other people to him. If the individual cannot elicit predictable reactions to his self presentation, then he cannot maintain a stable and consistent image of himself."[15]

Employees who seem involved in what is being said and done at meetings have a tendency to lean in on the table, and their bodily actions depict an involvement in the interactions that are taking place. On the other hand, bored group members have a tendency to lean away from the discussions taking place. Their bodily actions depict apathy and disinterest in what is being said and done. Nonverbal cues, such as body position and movement of the head, express the attitudes that we have, both positive and negative, and also reflect status relationships. Mehrabian believes that movements of the limbs and head indicate not only one's attitude toward a specific set of circumstances but also how dominant and how anxious one generally tends to be in social situations.[16]

A supervisor's bodily actions may be cues to let others know it is their turn to speak. Conversely, supervisors may send cues to others indicating that they would like to comment on what has just been said. In either case, supervisors, like everybody else, are constantly sending messages with their bodies.

Touching

Some everyday verbal expressions indicate the importance of touching in our daily lives: Keep in touch. He's a little touched. That really touched me. Don't be so touchy. That was a touching story. Nonverbal communication often creates a kind of intimacy seldom achieved by words alone.

In patient care, for example, nonverbal messages sent through touch often become an important way of communicating. Though eye contact is highly personalized, touching is the most intimate means of communicating through the senses. D.C. Aguilera, for example, found that touch behavior by nurses increased verbal output by patients and improved the patients' attitude toward the nurses.[17]

Seldom do we just compliment an employee on doing a good job. Most of the time the compliment is accompanied by a handshake, a pat on the back, or a slight squeeze of the arm. It is also interesting to note that it is usually the superior who has the right to initiate some aspect of touching.

The supervisor should also be aware, however, that touching is potentially the most threatening type of nonverbal behavior because it can degenerate into object-like control of other people. It can lead other persons to feel that they are being manipulated.

Conversely, when a supervisor's tactual contacts reflect genuine feelings, the employee feels confidence, acceptance, and encouragement—and responds accordingly.

The Use of Space

Space or distance not only communicates the intimacy of a relationship but is also used to communicate status. The first mention of space as a communicative variable is in the Gospel of Luke:

> When thou are invited to a wedding feast, do not recline in the first place, lest perhaps one more distinguished than thou have been invited by him. And he who had invited thee and him, come and say to thee, "Make room for this man" and then thou begin with shame to take the last place. But when thou art invited, go and recline in the last place; that when he who invited thee comes in, he may say to thee, "Friend go up higher!" Then thou wilt be honored in the presence of all who are at table with thee. For everyone who exalts himself shall be humbled, and he who humbles himself shall be exalted.[18]

Space communicates status. At some time or other, all of us have had bosses who sat and chatted with us on an office couch—until, that is, the subject turned to money or promotion, at which point they usually moved behind their desks and left us sitting alone on the couch. In this example, space can be seen as representing status that is highly personalized. All of us carry our personal space and status around with us as we stake out our territory within the limits of our influence.

Edward Hall believes that our use of space is communicative. How far people stand or sit from one another indicates how well they know one another and the purpose of their communication. Individuals send messages by placing themselves in certain spatial relationships with one another.[19]

This type of nonverbal behavior, called "proxemics," involves the relationships between the communicator's body and other people or objects in the environment. The next time you walk into your boss's office, look around and see what the room tells you. Can you walk directly into the office, or do you have to gain access through a secretary?

A.G. White reported on an experiment conducted in a physician's office. He found that a desk may significantly alter a patient's at-ease state. With the desk separating the patient and doctor, only 10 percent of the patients were perceived to be at ease. When the desk was removed, the at-ease state of the patients rose to 55 percent.[20]

Distance and space can tell supervisors things about their working relationships. When we like an employee, we stand rather close and might even touch them. In fact, try walking down a hospital corridor with someone you like without bumping shoulders. It's almost impossible. On the other hand, if you don't like someone, it is very easy to keep a proper distance and not bump shoulders.

A personnel director at a North Carolina hospital carried out an interesting experiment. He wrote on a piece of paper the people he worked with and felt close to. On the same paper he also wrote down the names of the people he worked with but didn't feel close to. Next he placed a chair by the door to his office, another chair in front of his desk, a third chair at the side of his desk, and a fourth one next to his own chair behind his desk. When people entered his office, he did not direct them to any specific chair. But after they left he wrote down where they had sat. As you might guess, he found out that those he felt closest to in his working relationships sat closest to him behind his desk; indeed some even sat in his own chair.

Julius Fast describes a set of experiments conducted by Robert Sommer, professor of psychology at the University of California:

> Dr. Sommer entered a hospital wearing a white doctor's coat, he then systematically invaded the patients' privacy, sitting next to them on benches, and entering their wards and day rooms. These intrusions, he reported, invariably bothered the patients and drove them from their special chairs or areas. The patients reacted to Dr. Sommer's physical intrusion by becoming uneasy and restless and finally by removing themselves from the area.[21]

Because personal space is invisible, people will tend to flee rather than fight if an intrusion is made into their space. Personal space can be thought of as a "plastic bubble" that surrounds the individual. When people meet, they position their bodies in such a way as to keep the walls of the bubbles intact. If one person pushes too close to another, the bubbles bounce apart.[22]

People, regardless of race or background, choose their spatial bubbles in light of their own values, mores, and cultures. When other people invade their personally created private zones, they become uncomfortable, aggressive, and sometimes even hostile.

According to Hall, there are three major interpersonal distances that govern our interpersonal relationships: (1) an intimate distance from 3 to 20 inches, (2) a social distance from 20 inches to 5 feet, and (3) a public distance from 5 feet to 100 feet.[23]

CULTURAL DISTANCES

In dealing with various ethnic groups it is important for supervisors to remember that the nonverbal behaviors of one group will not necessarily be the same as those of another group. Yet when nonverbal feedback is placed in its proper context, misinterpretations and misunderstandings between different culture groups can be reduced.

As noted by Hall, two to three feet from another person is a comfortable distance for most Americans for purposes of social conversation. In Brazil, Mexico, France, and most Arab countries, however, a comfortable distance for social conversation is somewhat shorter than two feet. Thus, in conversation the American is constantly moving back while a person from one of these other cultures is constantly moving forward.[24]

Here are some other differences in the behavior patterns of various cultural groups:

The Cultural Differences of Various Groups

Behavior Expressed	Behavior Pattern	Culture Group
Affection	Smelling heads	Mongols
	Rubbing noses	Eskimos
	Embracing or kissing	Eur-Americans
Approval	Smacking lips	Indians (N.A.)
	Backslapping	Eur-Americans
Assent	Elevating head	New Zealanders
	Nodding	Eur-Americans

Disrespect	Turning back	French
	Snapping finger under nose of opponent	Mediterraneans
Humility	Joining hands over head and bowing	Chinese
	Dropping arms, sighing	Europeans
	Bending body downward	Samoans
Salutation	Clapping hands	Loangoan people
	Waving of the hand	Eur-Americans

Source: George Brown, from an unpublished graduate paper (University of Denver, 1971).

We can see from this chart that nonverbal communicative behavior must be interpreted in its proper social context. These behaviors are culturally derived and thus must be learned by supervisors if they are to enjoy their maximum capacity to influence or adjust to various cultural environments.

Birdwhistell reinforces the point that there are no universal words, no sound complexes, that carry the same meaning the world over. There are no body actions, facial expressions, or gestures that provoke identical reactions in all countries.[25]

SUMMARY

As noted earlier, congruency between verbal and nonverbal messages helps to create clear, meaningful communication. However, not all message-sending is this simple. Even employee publications, at times, carry two messages. As Charles E. Redfield has observed, a company publication will often state that " 'people are our greatest asset,' but the front cover shows the new 500 million dollar building without an employee in sight. Or, it may say 'We are all one family,' but the material handler is shown in dirty dungarees and the general manager in a custom tailored suit."[26]

More could be said about nonverbal behavior for didactic purposes. The core problem, however, may be that, on the one hand, we are still struggling to conceptualize the key communication variable, information, while, on the other hand, we have too little knowledge of alternative ways of interpreting the various code systems available to people.

The art of nonverbal communication may be something like the statue of Venus de Milo; while interesting to look at, it still lacks the necessary hands to be called an effective *science*. Remember that, as you abstract nonverbal meaning from a message, you are merely making an educated guess with degrees of probability. If used properly with the right amount of discretion, nonverbal communication can be a useful tool that will enable you to discriminate more accurately in your search for common meaning.

NONVERBAL REVIEW PUZZLE

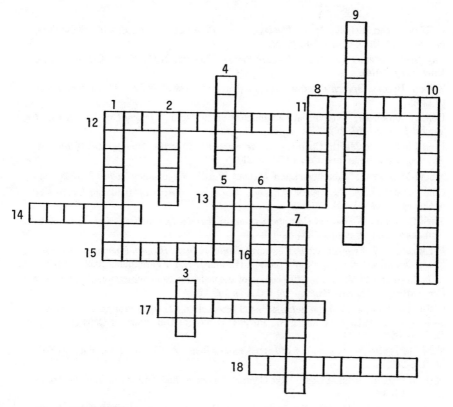

DOWN

1) An extension of self.
2) Most intimate of senses.
3) What you see is what you _____.
4) One's territory.
5) Number of minutes it takes to form a first impression.
6) Nonverbal interpretation depends upon this.
7) Harmonious verbal and nonverbal messages.
8) A kind of distance, from 20 inches to 5 feet.
9) Meaning derived from voice tone.
10) A highly personalized form of nonverbal communication (two words).

ACROSS

11) A form of communication.
12) How nonverbal messages are learned.
13) Expressions regarded as reliable indicators.
14) A kind of distance, from 5 to 100 feet.
15) A bodily action.
16) Number of basic types of messages sent at the same time.
17) We defend this.
18) The silent language.

(Answers are on page 112.)

NOTES

1. Gail Myers and Michelle Myers, *The Dynamics of Human Communication* (New York: McGraw-Hill Book Co., 1980), p. 203.

2. Ray Birdwhistell, *Paul Swain Lecture Series* (Raleigh, N.C.: North Carolina State University, 1974).

3. William Brooks, *Speech Communication* (Dubuque, Iowa: William C. Brown, 1974), p. 176.

4. Helmut Mossback, "Nonverbal Communication in Japan," *Journal of Nervous and Mental Disease* 157: 262-277.

5. Fred Fiedler and Martin Chemers, *Leadership and Effective Management* (Glenview, Ill.: Scott, Foresman and Co., 1974), p. 21.

6. Albert Mehrabian, "Communication Without Words," *Psychology Today* 2 (1968): 53.

7. Charles Darwin, *The Expression of Emotions in Man and Animals* (Chicago: University of Chicago Press, 1965).

8. Mark L. Knapp, *Nonverbal Communication in Human Interaction* (New York: Holt, Rhinehart, and Winston, 1972), p. 119.

9. P. Ekman, W.V. Friesen, and P. Ellsworth, *Emotion in the Human Face: Guidelines for Research and an Integration of Findings* (Elmford, N.Y.: Pergamon, 1962), p. 107.

10. A. Mehrabian and M. Weiner, "Decoding of Inconsistent Communications," *Journal of Personality and Social Psychology* 6 (1967): 109-114.

11. G. Simmel, "Sociology of the Senses: Visual Interaction," *Introduction to the Science of Sociology*, ed. R.E. Park and E.W. Burgess (Chicago: University of Chicago Press, 1921), p. 358.

12. Michael Argyle, *The Psychology of Interpersonal Behavior* (Baltimore: Penguin, 1967), pp. 115-116.

13. Michael Argyle and Janet Dean, "Eye Contact, Distance, and Affiliation," *Sociometry* 28 (1965): 289-304.

14. G. Myers and M. Myers, *The Dynamics of Human Communication* (New York: McGraw-Hill Book Co., 1973), p. 171.

15. Abne Eisenberg and Ralph Smith, *Nonverbal Communication* (New York: Bobbs-Merrill Co., 1971), pp. 66-67.

16. Albert Mehrabian, *Silent Messages* (Belmont, Calif.: Wadsworth Publishing Co., 1971), pp. 55-72.

17. D.C. Aguilera, "Relationships Between Physical Contact and Verbal Interaction Between Nurses and Patients," *Journal of Psychiatric Nursing* 5 (1967): 5-21.

18. Luke 14:1-11.

19. Edward Hall, *Hidden Dimensions* (Garden City, N.Y.: Doubleday & Co., 1966), pp. 1-6.

20. A.G. White, "The Patient Sits Down: A Clinical Note," *Psychosomatic Medicine* 15 (1953): 256-257.

21. Julius Fast, *Body Language* (New York: Pocket Books, 1961), pp. 45-46.

22. Robert Sommer, "Studies in Personal Space," *Sociometry* 22 (1959): 247-260.

23. Edward Hall, *Silent Language* (New York: Fawcett Premier Book, 1959), pp. 163-164.

24. Ibid.

25. Ray Birdwhistell, "Background to Kinesics," *Etc: A Review of General Semantics* 13 (1955): 10-18.

26. Charles E. Redfield, *Communication in Management* (Chicago: University of Chicago Press, 1958), pp. 141-142.

SUGGESTED READINGS

Argyle, Michael, and Dean, J. "Eye Contact, Distance and Affiliation," *Sociometry* 23: 289-304.

Birdwhistell, Ray. *Introduction to Kinesics.* Louisville: University of Louisville Press, 1970.

Casher, L., and Dixson, B.K. "The Therapeutic Use of Touch." *Journal of Psychiatric Nursing and Mental Health Services* 5: 442-451.

Ekman, P., and Friesen, W.V. "Head and Body Cues in the Judgment of Emotion: A Reformulation." *Perceptual and Motor Skills* 24: 711-724.

Felipe, N.J., and Sommer, R. "Invasions of Personal Space." *Social Problems* 14: 206-214.

Hall, Edward T. *The Silent Language.* Garden City, N.Y.: Doubleday & Co., 1959.

Knapp, Mark L. *Nonverbal Communication in Human Interaction.* New York: Holt, Rhinehart, and Winston, 1972.

Mahl, G.F. "Measuring the Patient's Anxiety During Interviews from Expressive Aspects of His Speech." *Transactions of the New York Academy of Sciences* 21: 249-257.

McCorkle, R. "Effects of Touch on Seriously Ill Patients." *Nursing Research* 23: 125-132.

Mehrabian, Albert. "Significance of Posture and Position in the Communication of Attitudes and Status Relationships." *Psychological Bulletin* 71: 359-372.

———. "Nonverbal Betrayal of Feeling." *Journal of Experimental Research in Personality* 5: 64-73.

———. "Communication Without Words." *Psychology Today* 2: 52-55.

Rosenfeld, H.M. "Approval Seeking and Approval Inducing Functions of Verbal and Non-verbal Responses in the Dyad." *Journal of Personality and Social Psychology* 4: 65-72.

Ruesch, J., and Kees, Weldon. *Nonverbal Communication.* Berkeley: University of California Press, 1956.

Sommer, Robert. *Personal Space: The Behavioral Basis of Design.* Englewood Cliffs, N.J.: Prentice Hall, 1969.

White, A.G. "The Patient Sits Down: A Clinical Note." *Psychosomatic Medicine* 15: 256-257.

Zaidel, S.F., and Mehrabian, A. "The Ability to Communicate and Infer Positive and Negative Attitudes Facially and Vocally." *Journal of Experimental Research in Personality* 3: 233-241.

NONVERBAL REVIEW PUZZLE

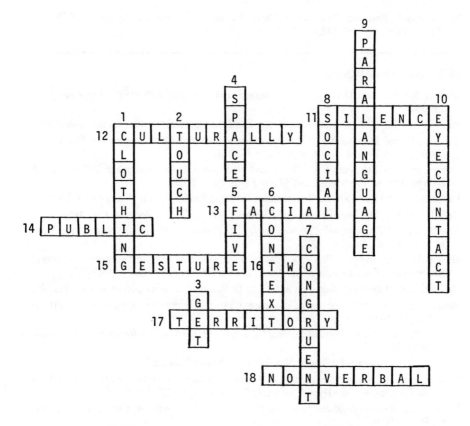

NONVERBAL REVIEW PUZZLE

DOWN

1) An extension of self.
2) Most intimate of senses.
3) What you see is what you _____.
4) One's territory.
5) Number of minutes it takes to form a first impression.
6) Nonverbal interpretation depends upon this.
7) Harmonious verbal and nonverbal messages.
8) A kind of distance, from 20 inches to 5 feet.
9) Meaning derived from voice tone.
10) A highly personalized form of nonverbal communication (two words).

ACROSS

11) A form of communication.
12) How nonverbal messages are learned.
13) Expressions regarded as reliable indicators.
14) A kind of distance, from 5 to 100 feet.
15) A bodily action.
16) Number of basic types of messages sent at the same time.
17) We defend this.
18) The silent language.

Chapter 7

The Dynamics of the Supervisor's Work Group

CHAPTER OBJECTIVES

The purpose of this chapter is to enable you to CHANGE your communicative behavior in a *positive* direction. After studying the material you should be able to:

Communicate more effectively in small groups.

Have an understanding of group dynamics.

Assess and improve communication flow between patients, coworkers, and employees.

Notice the differences between "supportive" and "defensive" group climates.

Gain new insights into the importance of group norms and roles.

Evaluate the quality of your work group in seven areas of group process.

INTRODUCTION

The health care industry today employs close to five million people and accounts for ten percent of our gross national product. The medical achievements are indeed impressive. Great progress has been made against a variety of diseases. Medical science has been able virtually to eliminate smallpox and polio. Rapid advances are being made in conquering cancer and heart disease. The health care community provides a service, but this service is only as good as the people who administer it. Few health care professionals work in isolation. Rather, health care demands coordination, not only between individuals but also between departments. No one department is more important than another. There is an interdependent need for support and communication exchange.

To enable this medical progress to continue, more sources of information have to be tapped and more people informed. Information must move through many channels before it reaches its intended destination. Intergroup communication affects many members of the health care team—the surgeon, anesthesiologist, nurse, comptroller, personnel staff, maintenance workers, payroll staff—indeed, every department within the organization. No organization can be productive without proper support personnel. This support, or the lack of it, will ultimately affect the health care organization's basic reason for existence—the care of the patient. Each health care group is dependent upon the goods or services provided by another group within the same organization. This interplay of groups determines the final outcome of success or failure.

SMALL GROUP CHARACTERISTICS

A group is a collection of individuals who affect the character of the group and who are in turn affected by the group. The same people might react differently in one group than they do in another group. Delete one member from a group and the group's character changes; add another member and it will change again. In each case, the varied combinations of individual interests, abilities, and personalities produce a different group behavior.

The characteristics of a group are determined by the people comprising that group. Individuals join groups to satisfy their personal needs, but the needs of one person are not necessarily the same as those of another person, either in kind or degree. Moreover, people change from moment to moment; a person who is cooperative at one moment may be hostile at another.

Dorwin Cartwright and Alvin Zander define a group of people as an informal psychological group when the members interact chiefly through oral communication. More explicitly, an informal psychological group is

- a collection of two or more individuals
- who consciously identify with one another and
- interact dynamically,
- chiefly through the medium of oral communication,
- in such a way that all members are utilized to meet the satisfaction needs of each.[1]

This working definition should not lead one to believe that only oral communication is used in small group interaction. The term *interacting dynamically* infers the use of nonverbal communication as a vital part of the group process.

THE DYNAMICS OF SMALL GROUPS

Sociologists and other theorists of small group interaction have discovered that small groups are highly task-oriented, usually operate under great pressure, and usually have rigidly controlled agendas. The members of these groups are constantly interacting dynamically. However, the dynamics can be either good or bad, depending upon the training and attitudes of the group members.

Harold P. Zelko refers to this interplay as a pattern of forces at work and lists ten elements that determine the group outcome:

1. the individual background of each member of the group
2. the status and position of each member
3. the emotional involvement of each member with the subject
4. the relationship of the members with each other
5. the status and position of the leader in relation to the members
6. the leader-group relationship in relation to the subject and outcome
7. the relative amount of leader and group participation

8. the relative amount and type of participation of each member
9. the effect of certain leadership methods and tools and the characteristics of the discussion
10. the effect of physical surroundings on the discussion[2]

Group Status

Each member of a group contributes status and prestige to the group and develops additional status and prestige within the group. Because of their status or prestige, certain employees assume responsibility for certain functions and are listened to more carefully by other group members.

Studies on member status within groups indicate that (1) high-status members tend to communicate more than low-status, (2) high-status members tend to communicate more with other high-status members, and (3) low-status members tend to communicate more with high-status members than with other low-status members.[3]

P.E. Slater discovered a high correlation between the rank of group members and the amount of talking they did within the group. High-status members gave the most information, received the most information, presented the best ideas, and gave guidance to the group's thinking.[4]

Group Norms

If rules are to be effective within a group, they must be accepted, and group members must know that they are accepted by others as well as by themselves. These conditions create a group norm, defined as "shared acceptance of a rule."[5]

The group leader plays an important role in establishing group norms. However, leaders cannot establish norms by themselves. Other high-status members help to influence new group norms or to reinforce norms that have been previously established. The high-status members also exert more influence upon group norms than do the average group members.

When individuals with deviant attitudes attempt to violate group norms, social pressures are exerted to bring them into line. Social pressure is highest in groups that are highly cohesive. Thus, if an employee expresses an opinion or uses language contrary to actions deemed acceptable, the group will concentrate its attention upon the employee with a barrage of comments until the employee gets back in line. If people insist upon deviating from the group norm, the group will give up on them and often ignore them entirely until they come around or get out of the group.

Group norms can be changed, but this is a difficult task. Usually, those who wish to change group norms must find support through changes in group personnel, in the excesses of established leaders, by external pressure for change, or through changes in the communication patterns of group members. Sometimes, a group feels it is time for self-evaluation and decides through deliberative group effort to change some of the existing group norms.

Dean Barnlund and Franklin Haiman conclude,

> at least on the basis of present knowledge, that those members of a group who have more authority than the others (the leader, senior members, etc.), those who have disturbed personalities, and those who happen to get attention first are more likely to be more influential in shaping group norms than the "average" member.[6]

Group Pressure

There is considerable evidence to indicate that individuals tend to conform to group standards, even when such standards contradict individual standards or beliefs. Solomon Asch conducted an experiment to examine the effect of group pressure on individual judgment. In each of his groups there were three trained subjects and one naive subject. All subjects were asked to judge which of two lines was longer. However, the trained subjects were instructed to say that the shorter line was longer. In most instances the trained subjects answered first, and then the naive subjects would go along with the majority view, regardless of their own perceptions.[7]

From this experiment it was generalized that in small groups the majority will tend to pull the minority to its point of view. Apparently, people need to belong to such an extent that they will sacrifice their own opinions for those of the group.

Group Size

A group's ability to reach decisions, derive group satisfaction, and communicate efficiently is dependent upon the size of the group. George Beal, Joe Bohlen, and J. Neil Raudabaugh believe that the optimum size for small group efficiency is five members:

(1) This size allows sufficient opportunity for each individual to participate and yet enough members are present to draw on content and make it worthwhile; (2) there is not the possibility of a strict deadlock as with even numbers; (3) if the group splits it tends to split into a majority of three and a minority of two, so that being in the minority it does not isolate any one individual; (4) the group seems large enough for members to shift roles easily . . . and allows a member to easily withdraw from an awkward position.[8]

Most authorities tend to think that, as group size increases beyond five members, there is less group cohesion, a greater tendency toward more formal procedures, and increased difficulty in coordinating activities; and the group leader tends to talk to the group as a whole rather than to individual group members.

Slater reports that members of five-man groups expressed complete satisfaction with the size of their groups, indicating that they were neither too large nor too small.[9]

As groups increase in size, subgroups form within the main group, and the number of interactions increases dramatically. This makes the task of structuring the group more difficult.

Robert Bostrom notes that in a dyad (two people) only two interactions are possible, A to B and B to A, but in a triad (three people) there are nine possibilities:[10]

A to B	B to C	A to B and C
A to C	C to B	B to A and C
B to A	C to A	C to A and B

He then shows the number of interactions that can take place in groups that range in size from two to eight members:[11]

Number in Group	Interactions Possible
2	2
3	9
4	28
5	75
6	186
7	441
8	1056

In summary, groups should be kept to a maximum working size of five members, if at all possible. If there is a need to increase the size of the group, it would be best to form subgroups of five members to increase efficiency and member satisfaction. It should also be remembered that size, like leadership, is dependent upon the situation. A supervisory work group, for example, may need to be larger than five. However, in general, five is the recommended size for a task-oriented, problem-solving group.

Group Setting

The setting in which employees discuss work problems and make organizational decisions is extremely important. The setting helps to establish the group climate, which we examined in detail in Chapter 2.

N.L. Mintz found that an "ugly" room produced different effects on people than a "beautiful" room. People in the beautiful room reported feelings of comfort and energy and a desire to continue the activity. People in the ugly room reported the opposite effects.[12]

A seating arrangement in a circular or elliptical pattern in which everyone can be seen and no one is in a physically dominant position may help to create a more open and friendly atmosphere.[13] Such a seating arrangement allows each employee in the group to see and respond to any other employee.

Barnlund concluded that eye contact is an important factor in spatial arrangements. In a study done in 1965, he found that, when interaction is desired, people seem to prefer to sit closer together and in a position in which eye contact is possible, rather than side by side, an arrangement that limits eye contact.[14]

The attractiveness of the room, type and intensity of lighting, ventilation, type of chairs, table size, and table shape all help to determine the type of work and communication that takes place within the small group.

During the Viet Nam War, the dispute over the size and shape of the negotiating table in Paris is a classic example of the importance placed on environmental factors as they symbolize status or equality.

James McCroskey describes this incident:

> The United States (US) and South Viet Nam (SVN) wanted a seating arrangement in which only two sides were identified. They did not want to recognize the National Liberation front (NLF) as an "equal" party in the

negotiations. North Viet Nam (NVN) and the NLF wanted "equal" status given to all parties—represented by a four sided table. The final arrangement was such that both parties could claim victory. The round table minus the dividing lines allowed North Viet Nam and the NLF to claim all four delegations were equal. The existence of the two secretarial tables (interpreted as dividers), the lack of identifying symbols on the table, and an AA, BB speaking rotation permitted the United States and South Viet Nam to claim victory for the two sided approach. Considering the amount of lives lost during the eight months needed to arrive at the seating arrangement, we can certainly conclude that territorial space has extremely high priority in some interpersonal settings.[15]

Group Goals

Many organizations have goals, but often the goals are unclear, nebulous, or unrealistic. Employees must accept group goals in order for the group to achieve success, but the goals must also be closely related to the needs of the individual group members. Bobby Patton and Kim Giffin believe that the importance of goal specificity cannot be overemphasized. Their work has led them to conclude that groups fail, lose member commitment, bog down, and develop interpersonal dislikes because of a lack of specific goal identification.[16] Their point is that, if you aim for nothing in particular, it is likely you will achieve just that.

COMMUNICATION NETWORKS

The four main communication networks employed by organizations and small groups are represented by the following figures:

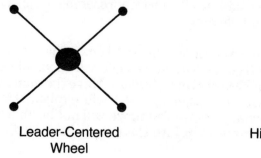

Leader-Centered
Wheel

Hierarchical
Chain

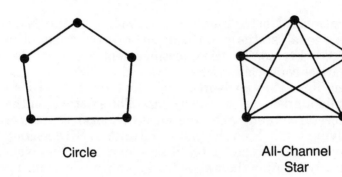

Circle

All-Channel
Star

The Wheel

The wheel network allows the central person to communicate with any group member, and in turn the members must direct all their comments through the center. Harold Leavitt discovered that the central person in the wheel usually becomes the leader and enjoys that position much more than those on the periphery enjoy their positions.[17]

Harold Guetzkow and Herbert A. Simon discovered that the wheel, while efficient in its use of time, tends to lower the cohesiveness of the group, reduce its inventiveness, and make its members too dependent upon the leader.[18]

The Chain

One of the major weaknesses of the chain communication network is that, as a message is passed from one person to the next, distortion takes place, some information is lost, and some information is added. Each person in the chain interprets the message somewhat differently and passes on the new interpretation. When the message reaches the end of the chain, it often barely resembles the original message. Consider the following:

- The colonel to the executive officer: "Tomorrow evening at approximately 2000 hours, Halley's comet will be visible in this area, an event that occurs every 75 years. Have the men fall out in the battalion area in fatigues, and I will explain this rare phenomenon to them. In case of rain, we will not be able to see anything, so march the men into the theatre and I will show them films of it."

- The executive officer to the company commander: "By order of the colonel, tomorrow at 2000 hours, Halley's comet will appear above the battalion area. If it rains, fall the men out in fatigues, then march to the theatre where the rare phenomenon will take place, something which occurs every 75 years."

- The company commander to the lieutenant: "By order of the colonel in fatigues at 2000 hours tomorrow evening, the phenomenal Halley's comet will appear in the theatre. In case of rain in the battalion area, the colonel will give another order, something which occurs every 75 years."

- The lieutenant to the sergeant: "Tomorrow at 2000 hours the colonel will appear in the theatre with Halley's comet, something which happens every 75 years if it rains. The colonel will then order the comet into the battalion area."

- The sergeant to the squad: "When it rains tomorrow at 2000 hours, the phenomenal 75-year-old General Halley, accompanied by the colonel, will drive his comet through the battalion area theatre in fatigues."

In Downward Communication

The chain is used by organizations primarily for downward communication. This enables top management to send messages to its employees. Obviously, there is a need for this type of communication network. Yet, as we have noted, the chain does have serious limitations. Research studies tend to indicate that much of the downward flow of information, from management to employees, is filtered out, distorted, or forgotten when the employees feel the information is not relevant to their needs and interests.

Helen Baker, John W. Ballentine, and John M. True discovered in their survey of company and union communication at the Bayway refinery of Esso Standard Oil Co. that "where it is direct and pertinent the information makes a lasting impression; where it is not, it is apt to be passed over and forgotten quickly."[19]

Bill Conboy reports on the percentage of information lost as the message moves from its point of dissemination, the board of directors, to its destination, the company employees:[20]

- Board of Directors ....100% of communication content retained
- Vice-Presidents .... 67% '' '' '' ''
- Supervisors .... 56% '' '' '' ''
- Managers .... 40% '' '' '' ''
- Foremen .... 30% '' '' '' ''
- Workers .... 20% '' '' '' ''

In Upward Communication

In his RAND Corporation monograph, Anthony Downs states that communication distortion takes place not only in a downward pattern but in an upward pattern as well. Subordinates will facilitate upward-directed messages that they believe will either please the boss or enhance their own welfare. On the other hand, superiors will suppress messages directed to subordinates if they perceive such messages as having a deleterious effect upon themselves or the organization.[21]

This conclusion is supported by P. Krivonos, who surveyed the findings of upward-communication research and concluded:

- Subordinates tend to distort information upward in a manner that pleases their superiors.

- Subordinates tend to tell their superiors what they want them to know.

- Subordinates tend to tell their superiors what they think they want to hear.

- Subordinates tend to tell their superiors information that reflects favorably on themselves and/or does not reflect negatively on themselves.[22]

The Circle

The circle network lends itself to high participation and usually results in high group member satisfaction. At times, however, frustration can occur due to the fact that there is no central source of information. The circle tends to promote equality among all group members. No one member has a position of authority that reduces intra-group status. The circle encourages high member participation.

The Star

Most authorities agree that, in the majority of cases, the star pattern is the most suitable. The star pattern, also called the all-channel network, allows anyone to talk to any other group member at any time. This allows direct communication to obtain necessary information. Moreover, the star can be easily rearranged to fit the internal needs of the group for varying types of information flow. Finally, member satisfaction appears to be highest in the star network.

Gerald Goldhaber examined communication patterns in a sample of almost 4,000 employees in 16 organizations in the United States and Canada. He discovered

- The farther up the organizational hierarchy an employee is, the less the followup regarding information sent to top management and in response to requests.

- The best sources of information are persons closest to the employees (coworkers, immediate supervisors); the worst sources are persons farthest away (top management, the boss's boss, formal management presentations).

- Information from top management is of lower quality than that from other key sources.

- The immediate communication climate is healthier than that of the organization at large (which limits openness, lacks sufficient incentives and rewards, and minimizes input, influence, and advancement opportunities).[23]

SUMMARY

Marvin Shaw summarized the findings of 18 communication networks and concluded that "the wheel and the chain are better when the problem is simple. . . . However, when the problem is complex the decentralized networks such as the circle and star are faster, more accurate, and result in higher member satisfaction."[24]

The research on communication networks continually points to one key variable that seems to determine the clarity and impact of the message sent. That key variable is distance, or how far removed the receiver is from the source of the original message. The circle and the star place the sender and receiver of messages in closer proximity to one another, which tends to facilitate retention and clarity during the communication exchange.

SMALL GROUP REVIEW PUZZLE

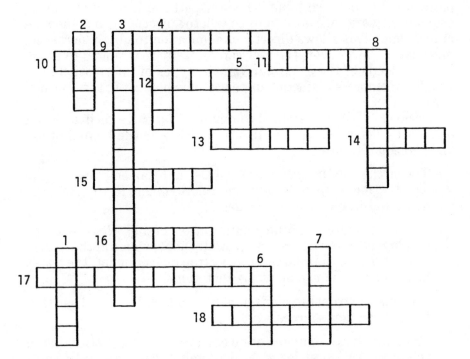

DOWN

1) A group must have these.
2) What status do members have who present the best ideas?
3) Effective groups have a high degree of this.
4) Number of people in a triad.
5) Affects the ability of groups to reach decisions.
6) The best type of network for most purposes.
7) A hierarchical network.
8) A group's environmental conditions.

ACROSS

9) Affected by group decisions.
10) Ideal group size.
11) One's position in a group.
12) Specific types of individual behavior exhibited by a group member.
13) Every group needs one of these.
14) Number of possible interactions in a group of eight people.
15) A network with no central source of information.
16) Shared acceptance of a rule.
17) Group togetherness.
18) One type of group.

(Answers are on page 129.)

NOTES

1. Dorwin Cartwright and Alvin Zander, *Group Dynamics* (New York: Harper & Row Publishers, 1968), pp. 46-48.

2. Harold P. Zelko, *Successful Discussion and Conference Techniques* (New York: McGraw-Hill Book Co., 1957), pp. 14-15.

3. J.I. Hurwitz, A.F. Zander, and B. Hymovitch, "Some Effects of Power on the Relationships Among Group Members," *Group Dynamics*, ed. D. Cartwright and A. Zander (New York: Harper & Row, Publishers, 1968), pp. 291-297.

4. P.E. Slater, "Role Differentiation in Small Groups," *American Sociological Review* 20 (1955): 303.

5. Theodore M. Newcomb, Ralph H. Turner, and Phillip E. Converse, *Social Psychology* (New York: Holt, Rhinehart, and Winston, Inc., 1965), p. 254.

6. Dean C. Barnlund and Franklin S. Haiman, The Dynamics of Discussion (Boston: Houghton Mifflin Co., 1960), pp. 199-200.

7. Solomon E. Asch, "Effects of Group Pressure Upon the Modification and Distortion of Judgments," *Readings in Social Psychology*, ed. G. Swanson et al. (New York: Holt, Rhinehart, and Winston, 1952), pp. 2-11.

8. George M. Beal, Joe M. Bohlen, and J. Neil Raudabaugh, *Leadership and Dynamic Group Actions* (Ames, Iowa: Iowa State University Press, 1962), pp. 117-118.

9. P.E. Slater, "Contrasting Correlates of Group Size," *Sociometry* 21 (1958): 129-139.

10. Robert Bostrom, "Patterns of Communicative Interaction in Small Groups," *Speech Monographs* 37 (1970): 257.

11. Ibid., p. 258.

12. N.L. Mintz, "Effects of Esthetic Surroundings: II. Prolonged and Repeated Experience in a 'Beautiful' and 'Ugly' Room." *Journal of Psychology* 41 (1956): 459-466.

13. Beal, Bohlen, and Raudabaugh, *Leadership and Dynamic Group Actions*, p. 81.

14. Dean C. Barnlund, *Interpersonal Communication: Survey and Studies* (Boston: Houghton Mifflin Co., 1968), pp. 559-560.

15. James McCroskey, Carl E. Larson, and Mark L. Knapp, *An Introduction to Interpersonal Communication* (Englewood Cliffs, N.J.: Prentice Hall, Inc., 1971), p. 97.

16. Bobby R. Patton and Kim Giffin, *Problem Solving Group Interaction* (New York: Harper & Row Publishers, 1973), pp. 147-148.

17. Harold Leavitt, "Some Effects of Certain Communication Patterns on Group Performance," *Journal of Abnormal and Social Psychology* 46 (1951): 38-50.

18. Harold Guetzkow and Herbert A. Simon, "The Impact of Certain Communication Nets Upon Organization and Performance in Task-Oriented Groups," *Management Science* 1 (1955): 233-250.

19. Helen Baker, John W. Ballentine, and John M. True, *"Transmitting Information Through Management and Union Channels: Two Case Studies.* Research report series no. 78 (Princeton: N.J.: Industrial Relations Section, Princeton University, 1949), p. 103.

20. Bill Conboy, *Working Together: Communication in a Healthy Organization* (Columbus, Ohio: Charles E. Merrill Publishing Co., 1976), p. 27.

21. Anthony Downs, *Inside Bureaucracy* (Santa Monica, Calif.: Rand Corporation, 1964), pp. 118-123.

22. P. Krivonos, "Distortion of Subordinate to Superior Communication" (Paper presented at a meeting of the International Communication Association, Portland, Ore., 1976).

23. Gerald M. Goldhaber, *Organizational Communication* (Dubuque, Iowa: William C. Brown Company, Publishers, 1979), p. 176.

24. Marvin E. Shaw, "Communication Networks," *Advances in Experimental Social Psychology*, vol. 1, ed. Leonard Berkowitz (New York: Academic Press, 1964), pp. 111-147.

SUGGESTED READINGS

Applbaum, Ronald L.; Bodaken, Edward M.; Sereno, Kenneth K.; and Anatol, Karl. *The Process of Group Communication*. Chicago: Science Research Associates, Inc., 1979.

Aronoff, Joel, and Messe, Lawrence A. "Motivational Determinants of Small Group Structure." *Journal of Personality and Social Psychology* 17: 319-324.

Bales, Robert F. *Interaction Process Analysis*. Reading, Mass.: Addison-Wesley, 1950.

Bavelas, A. "Communication Patterns in Task Oriented Groups." *Journal of Acoustical Society of America* 22: 725-730.

Bradford, Leland P. *Group Development*. La Jolla, Calif.: University Associates, Inc., 1974.

Cartwright, Dorwin, and Zander, Alvin, eds. *Group Dynamics*. New York: Harper & Row, Publishers, 1968.

Combs, A.W.; Avila, D.L.; and Purkey, W.W. *Helping Relationships Basic Concepts for the Helping Professions*. Boston: Allyn and Bacon, 1971.

Conboy, Bill. *Working Together: Communication in a Healthy Organization*. Columbus, Ohio: Charles E. Merrill Publishing Company, 1976.

Hare, Paul A., and Larson, Carl E. "Seating Position and Small Group Interaction." *Sociometry* 26: 480-486.

Jacobs, Alfred, ed. *The Group as Agent of Change*. New York: Human Science Press, 1974.

Leth, Pamela C., and Vandemark, JoAnn F. *Small Group Communication*. Menlo Park, Calif.: Cummings Publishing Co., Inc., 1977.

Pfeiffer, J. William, and Jones, John E. *A Handbook of Structured Experiences for Human Relations Training*, vols. 1-6. Iowa City, Iowa: University Associates Press, 1973-1977.

Phillips, Gerald M., and Erickson, Eugene C. *Interpersonal Dynamics in the Small Group*. New York: Random House, 1970.

Roberts, K.H., and O'Reilly, C.A. "Failures in Upward Communication in Organizations: Three Possible Culprits." *Academy of Management Journal* 17: 205-215.

Rosenfeld, H., and Rosenfeld A. *Human Interaction in the Small Group Setting*. Columbus, Ohio: Charles E. Merrill Publishing Co., 1973.

Sattler, William M., and Miller, N. Edd. *Discussion and Conference*. Englewood Cliffs, N.J.: Prentice Hall, Inc., 1968.

Schien, E.H., and Bennis, W.G. *Personal and Organizational Change Through Group Methods*. New York: John Wiley and Sons, 1965.

SMALL GROUP REVIEW PUZZLE

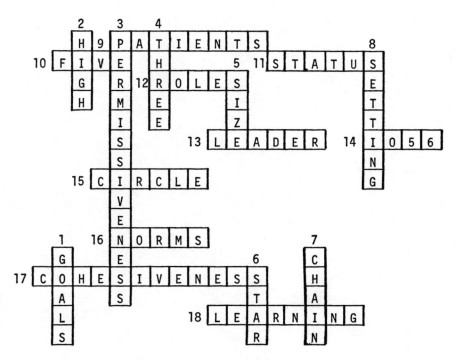

	DOWN		ACROSS

DOWN

1) A group must have these.
2) What status do members have who present the best ideas?
3) Effective groups have a high degree of this.
4) Number of people in a triad.
5) Affects the ability of groups to reach decisions.
6) The best type of network for most purposes.
7) A hierarchical network.
8) A group's environmental conditions.

ACROSS

9) Affected by group decisions.
10) Ideal group size.
11) One's position in a group.
12) Specific types of individual behavior exhibited by a group member.
13) Every group needs one of these.
14) Number of possible interactions in a group of eight people.
15) A network with no central source of information.
16) Shared acceptance of a rule.
17) Group togetherness.
18) One type of group.

Chapter 8

The Effectiveness of the Supervisor's Work Group

CHAPTER OBJECTIVES

The purpose of this chapter is to enable you to CHANGE your communicative behavior in a *positive* direction. After studying the material you should be able to:

Conduct meetings more efficiently.

Help your employees make better use of meeting time.

Assess the effectiveness of your work group.

Notice hidden agendas when they arise in meetings.

Generate more participation during group meetings and conferences.

Encourage participative decision making.

The biggest trouble with industry is that it is full of human beings. The longer you are president, the more firmly that fact will be riveted in your mind. That is why you will lose sleep. That is why your hair will turn gray, then get thin, and then fall out altogether, unless you are lucky. You will learn to your sorrow that, while a drill press never sulks and a drop hammer never gets jealous of other drop hammers, the same cannot be said for people. You will learn that a turret lathe may run one part for 10 years without affecting its ability or its willingness to be switched at any time to another part. But men are not that way. They develop habits and likes and dislikes.

You will learn that you have with people the same general problems of preventative maintenance, premature obsolescence, and complete operational failure that you have with machines. Only they are much harder to solve.

John L. McCaffrey, President
International Harvester Company

INTRODUCTION

Yes, at times, people seem to get in the way and make the task at hand more difficult rather than easier. As a supervisor, however, you are in the *people* business. People are all you have to work with, and it takes people to get the job done. This requires that supervisors coordinate task assignments, impart information, and exchange ideas with their work groups. Much of this supervisory instruction takes place through the use of meetings and small group conferences.

THE USE OF MEETINGS

Harold P. Zelko and Frank Dance believe that there are five current trends that account for the increased use of meetings and conferences:

1. The trend toward a more social-interacting work climate. We have become so specialized in our vocations that we are interdependent upon one another. Consultations and conferences are an essential part of just doing our jobs.

2. The trend toward giving more participative opportunities to employees to express themselves and be heard and to have a voice in matters that concern them. This puts the conference in a dominant position as a major forum for such opportunities.
3. The trend toward more consultation with subordinates, now characterized as consultative management. This means increasing reliance on the conference setting for drawing out the opinions and judgments of members of a work group.
4. The trend toward reliance on group decision making by anyone who supervises the work of others. This has a direct effect on the extent to which the conference method is used.
5. The trend toward democratic management. This puts the group-leader relationship strongly in focus.[1]

Meetings can be a useful tool and indeed are essential in imparting or gaining information. They are also the best means of sharing or solving common problems. At times, meetings may be regarded as a cure-all for all organizational problems. At other times, the feeling may be that we really have no need for a meeting, except for the fact that it's Tuesday, and we always have a meeting on Tuesday. Yet, the fact is that much of our time is spent in meetings.

R. Tillman found that 94 percent of organizations with more than 10,000 employees have formal committees.[2] M. Kriesberg reported that executives typically spend an average of 10 hours a week in formal committee meetings.[3] A survey conducted by Executive Standards, a management consulting firm, and reported by Connecticut General Life Insurance Company in 1975, showed that the average executive spends almost 7,000 hours a year in meetings. That averages out to almost two out of five working days.[4]

Stewart Tubbs reports that

> . . . one Ford Motor Company division improved their meetings by requiring committee members to report in writing to the division general manager any meeting lasting over one hour. In addition, each member was encouraged to indicate whether he or she thought the meeting was worth the time involved. This plan resulted in shorter meetings, better agendas, and an increased sense of responsibility on the part of the committee chairperson.[5]

BEHAVIORS THAT DECREASE MEETING EFFECTIVENESS

In any meeting that involves a group of employees there will be present power relationships; that is, one person will have influence over another within that group. The mere existence of such a power relationship can and does, at times, pose a threat to the employee being influenced, and we should expect that employee to seek ways of defending against it.

Jack Gibb has developed six categories of behavior that arouses defensiveness and ultimately affects the climate of the meeting or conference.

1. *Evaluation:* to question a person's values, standards, or motives. Even the simplest question may evoke defensiveness. Once, at a meeting, a colleague replied to a statement of one of the authors by saying, "Well, Harry, there are some of us who are professional enough to feel. . . ." Well, that reply produced an immediate defensive reaction, because the statement strongly suggested that the author was not professional. Employees need to question, yet only through a supportive climate of trust will they feel free to question policy or instructions. Questioning allows an employee the opportunity to learn and grow and thus become more competent. An employee can be supportive by presenting feelings, events, perceptions, or processes that do not ask or imply that other employees change their behaviors or attitudes. Our questions should be genuine requests for information.

2. *Control:* to try to do something to another person to change that person's attitude or belief. If hidden motives are suspected, resistance is increased. Other group members can overcome this resistance by showing a desire to collaborate in defining a mutual problem and in seeking its solution.

3. *Strategy:* to make others think they are making their own decisions, to make them feel that the speaker has a genuine interest in them. No one likes to be the victim of hidden motivation. Employees in staff meetings should look for a speaker's remarks that reflect spontaneity rather than manipulation. They should communicate with those who respond spontaneously and in a straightforward, honest manner.

4. *Neutrality:* to express lack of concern for a fellow group member, to be clinical or detached from the feelings of the group. Neutrality suggests indifference, and indifference

breeds contempt. To solve common problems and share ideas, group members must develop rapport with their colleagues.

5. *Superiority:* to communicate one's status as superior. For a group to be effective, its members must have a feeling of equality (no other member's ideas are better than mine) and must work together on an equal basis to solve common problems.

6. *Certainty:* to assume you have all the right answers. Employees should develop attitudes of patience and try to avoid frozen judgments until all the evidence has been presented. Medical procedures are not employed until all the diagnostic tests have been taken and analyzed. The same should be true of group decision making. Group members should be allowed to have their say and then, based on that information, an opinion may be formed.[6]

A further note might be made regarding a person's tendency to become defensive. A common rejoinder to this tendency is that "you're getting defensive!" This reply strongly suggests that there is something wrong with being defensive. If a person became defensive over every remark made in that person's direction, one might have reason to question the person's emotional state. In many instances, however, we have a right to become defensive. We should defend the things we believe in. Indeed, sometimes a little anger and a red face can show dramatically where we stand on a particular issue. In fact, such instances may represent the few times that we are communicating with complete clarity.

In any meeting you will like some of your colleagues more than others. There may even be present a few colleagues whom you do not like at all. This brings to mind an ancient verse:

> I do not like thee, Dr. Fell,
>   And why it is I cannot tell.
> But this I know and know full well—
>   I do not like thee, Dr. Fell.[7]

Sometimes our personal dislike for a fellow group member creates a hidden agenda that keeps the group from reaching its full potential. At such times, we must make a concerted effort to remain objective, to treat those that we are not too fond of with, at least, some semblance of professional dignity.

Richard Huseman, James Lahiff, and John Hatfield have found that hidden agendas severely limit group productivity:

Hidden agenda are comprised of the personal attitudes and emotions of an individual. Unlike the agenda for a meeting that is apparent to all of the participants, an individual's hidden agenda may remain unnoticed for any number of meetings. A person's hidden agenda may be his ulterior motives for having joined the group, or his desire to make another group member look bad. Such a hidden agenda may retard the progress of the group until it is given a full airing. Since such agenda often remain unverbalized and other members obviously remain oblivious to them, feelings of frustration may envelop the group and further limit its accomplishments as well as weaken its ties.[8]

Communication Stoppers

Most supervisors are aware of the advantages of group brainstorming. In such situations, no idea is ridiculous; quantity, not quality, is wanted; and everyone attempts to capitalize on the ideas of others. Eventually, the best ideas are selected and refined from those that have been presented.

However, whether the group is brainstorming or only one person is expressing a new idea, the effort may be hampered by "communication stoppers." Lester R. Bittel cites the following communication stoppers:

- "That's ridiculous."
- "We tried that before."
- "That will never work."
- "That's crazy."
- "It's too radical a change."
- "We're too small for that."
- "It's not practical."
- "Let's get back to reality."
- "You can't teach an old dog new tricks."
- "We'll be the laughing stock."

- "You're absolutely wrong."
- "You don't know what you're talking about."
- "It's impossible."
- "There's no way it can be done."[9]

These types of responses discourage group members from presenting new or different ideas. Ideas in meetings should flow freely. They should be seen as attempts to help the group meet its goal or resolve the issue being discussed. Supervisors often ask why their employees don't participate more in group meetings, why the same group members dominate every meeting. In a survey, Franklin Haiman asked his least talkative students why they did not actively participate in class discussions. He discovered the following 18 motives for nonparticipation. These motives seem to apply to all groups, not merely those in an academic setting:

1. A lack of confidence in one's own ideas: "It doesn't make any difference whether I say anything or not, because I never have anything original to contribute."
2. A lack of emotional involvement in the matters being discussed: "I just don't feel excited about the subject."
3. A lack of skill in verbalizing ideas: "The others can state their ideas so much more clearly than I can; so I'd rather just listen."
4. An inability to think rapidly enough to keep up with the pace of the discussion: "By the time I have mulled over a point long enough to have something to say on it, the rest of the group has moved on to something else."
5. A deeper reflection of ideas: "Some people just seem to think out loud, but I prefer to think to myself a while before speaking."
6. An attitude of detached observation: "I just like to hear what other people have to say about things."
7. Habitual shyness: "I never talk very much."
8. A lack of sleep or other physical disturbances: "I could hardly keep my eyes open."
9. Distraction of more pressing personal problems: "The reason I didn't talk today was that I was worrying about a midterm exam I have next period."

10. Submissiveness to more aggressive members: "A guy can never get a word in edgewise in this outfit, so I just keep quiet."
11. An interpersonal conflict: "I knew that if I ever got started I would have told that _____ off, so I decided not to say anything at all."
12. A nonpermissive atmosphere: "I don't feel free to speak when Miss _____ is around."
13. An overdominant leader: "He doesn't care what I think. He just wants an audience to make big speeches."
14. Fear of being rejected: "I'm afraid that everybody will think that what I have to say is silly."
15. A solidified pattern of participation: "Everybody in the group has gotten used to my not talking much, so I feel uncomfortable—as though everyone were surprised—when I do speak."
16. A feeling of superiority: "That was such a pointless discussion and no one really knew what they were talking about. What a waste of time."
17. A disbelief in the value of the discussion: "Talk never changes anybody's mind, so why bother."
18. Lack of knowledge or intelligence: "The discussion was way over my head."[10]

Supervisors should be especially aware of the pattern of communication that solidifies within groups. This awareness can help them to construct a better communicative balance among the group members. In most psychology texts, this solidified pattern is referred to as the "communicative pecking order," because the process is similar to the pecking order of chickens at feeding time, that is, one chicken eats first, followed by a second, and so on.

Thus, at the start of a meeting, the employee who speaks first can greatly influence the standards of the group. The initial comment of that employee may stimulate comments from others, and, before the group is aware of what has happened, group standards of participation have been established. On the other hand, the longer an employee waits to contribute an idea or to share information, the more difficult it becomes for that employee to speak and to influence the group. Observe your work group and see if a speaking order has been established in it.

Such a speaking order is not necessarily harmful; in some instances, however, good ideas from the more reluctant group members might as a result be overlooked.

BEHAVIORS THAT INCREASE MEETING EFFECTIVENESS

Supervisors are constantly involved with employees who either tend to dominate meetings or who are reluctant and keep their participation to the minimal accepted level. These two differing types of personalities must be dealt with if meetings are to be effective. Carl Heyel has identified a number of characteristics of such individuals and suggests ways of dealing with them:

- *Overly-talkative:* A show off, eager beaver, or just plain gabby. Cut across with a summarizing statement and direct a question to someone else.

- *Highly argumentative:* A combative personality, a professional heckler, or someone upset by emotional problems. Try to find merit in one of the person's points and get agreement on it, then move on to something else. Try to apply the process of conciliation. As a last resort, talk to the person privately after the meeting and see if you can get the person's cooperation for future meetings.

- *Quick-helpful:* One who has the right answers but keeps others out. Cut across tactfully by questioning others, for example: "Let's get several options." Use the person to summarize, but be sure you make clear your appreciation for the person's help.

- *Rambler:* One who talks about everything except the subject, one who gets lost. When the person stops for breath, extend thanks, rephrase one of the person's statements, and move on. Ask direct questions of others. Indicate in a friendly manner that the person is off the topic.

- *Side conversationalist:* Someone whose talk may be related but is distracting. Pause and let others listen; the comments may be pertinent. Call the person by name, then draw the person into the discussion by asking for his or her opinion.

- *Poor voice or choice of words:* One whose voice is not clear, who can't find the right words; one whose ideas may be good but who can't convey them. Repeat the person's ideas in your own words, but say, "Let me repeat that," rather than, "What you mean is. . . ." Protect the person from ridicule.

- *Obstinate:* One who won't budge, who has prejudices, or who simply may not see the point. Try to get others to help the person see the point. If time is short, tell the person frankly that it is necessary to get on with the meeting.

- *Griper:* Someone with a pet peeve, a professional griper, or one who may have a legitimate complaint. Explain that the problem is how to operate under the present system. Direct attention to the topic under discussion. Indicate the pressure of time.

- *Wrong subject:* Someone who is off the beam. Direct attention to topic under discussion, for example: "Something I said may have thrown you off the subject, but the question we are considering now is. . . ."

- *Definitely wrong:* One who is completely off the beam. Explain that "that's one way of looking at it," and go on. Ask additional questions, such as, "Would we be able to reconcile that with . . . ?" but don't embarrass the person.

- *Personality clash:* Two or more members in confrontation. Emphasize points of agreement as much as possible. Cut across with a direct question on the topic. Bring a disinterested member into the discussion. Ask that personalities be left out.

- *Superior attitude:* One not disposed to help, one whose attitude is, "I had to find out the hard way, son, you do the same." Explain that the meeting is a cooperative effort. Flatter the person by emphasizing how much the others could benefit by that person's experience. Don't overdo it, or the group will resent it.

- *Won't talk:* A person who is bored, indifferent, hesitant, insecure, or afraid. Try to determine the person's motivation and interest. Call on the person to relate an experience or opinion. Use direct, provocative questions; ask for agreement. Ask direct questions that you are sure the person can answer; be complimentary and sincere. If the person is seated near you, ask for the person's opinion to convey the impression that the person is talking to you rather than to the group.[11]

If groups are to resolve problems, plan, and make decisions, it is imperative that the group members' personality traits be effectively dealt with. This means that the supervisor must strive to be flexible while still being fair. The supervisor must involve the group in the decision-making process.

Considerable research has focused on the effects of active and passive participation in the making of a decision and on the levels of commitment to the decision once it has been reached. These studies indicate that individuals are more committed to a decision, have better attitudes toward the decision, and are more likely to follow through in implementing it when they are involved in the decision-making process.[12]

WORK GROUP MEMBERS NEED NOT ALWAYS AGREE

At times, supervisors think they have extremely effective work groups because the group members seldom disagree with one another's opinions. Research indicates, however, that group members can disagree without being disagreeable or damaging the effectiveness of the group.

Paul E. Torrence examined the effectiveness of air crews in combat during the Korean War. He concluded that

> . . . the more effective crews . . . were characterized by greater tolerance of disagreement. Several studies support the contention that the more effective groups are characterized by greater participation, initially wider divergence of expressed judgment, and greater acceptance of decisions. Not only was the quality found to be better as freedom of dissent increased, but the group tended to arrive at a higher degree of consensus, which in turn also appeared to be related to combat effectiveness of bomber crews.[13]

Too often, we associate opposition or disagreement in meetings with personal dislike. Yet, just because people oppose our ideas or disagree with us does not necessarily mean they dislike us. In 500 B.C., Confucius showed that opposition is the natural prerequisite for union. He noted that "as a result of opposition, a need to bridge it arises; this is true of all things, heaven and earth, man and woman. It is the individual differences between things that enable us to differentiate between them and this helps us to ultimately resolve those differences."[14]

Bobby R. Patton and Kim Giffin note that disagreement on the nature of the problem or the value of a suggested solution is a necessary component of the process of group interaction, but that perceived personal dislike creates a negative, debilitating response.

It is essential to discriminate accurately between disagreement and personal dislike if we are going to solve problems cooperatively.[15]

The following questionnaire will help you to examine your perceptions, related to your work group's effectiveness, in seven group-process areas.

GROUP EFFECTIVENESS QUESTIONNAIRE

This questionnaire examines your personal perception of the effectiveness of your work group, whether you are doing your job individually or working with other group members to meet a group goal. The questionnaire deals with seven parts of the group process: planning, problem solving/ decision making, use of resources, responsibility, motivation/pride, communications, and climate.

Each part may be scored separately to determine the group's strength or weakness in each of the process areas. The combined scores give a total group effectiveness score. Score each statement as follows: 1 = Strongly disagree. 2 = Disagree. 3 = Don't know or neutral. 4 = Agree. 5 = Strongly agree. The evaluative categories of the combined scores are shown at the end of the questionnaire.

Planning	*Disagree*			*Agree*	
(1) Our group goals are clearly defined.	1	2	3	4	5
(2) There is a high degree of commitment toward group goals.	1	2	3	4	5
(3) My group sets high standards of performance.	1	2	3	4	5
(4) The group does advance planning to avoid a crisis-like operating style.	1	2	3	4	5
(5) Our goals are well coordinated with other associated work groups and with higher organizational goals.	1	2	3	4	5
(6) Management asks for my ideas about better planning.	1	2	3	4	5
(7) When procedural changes are made or new equipment is placed in operation, my group is properly trained and prepared.	1	2	3	4	5
(8) Management provides adequate staffing.	1	2	3	4	5

Problem Solving/Decision Making	*Disagree*			*Agree*	
(9) My group develops several options before proposing a solution to a problem.	1	2	3	4	5
(10) In resolving group problems, each member of our group accepts a responsibility and constructively works toward resolution.	1	2	3	4	5
(11) We quickly resolve operational problems so that personal conflict does not build up.	1	2	3	4	5
(12) There is a general satisfaction concerning the quality of operational decisions that affect our group.	1	2	3	4	5
(13) Management accepts the consequences of a wrong decision and does not pass the blame to subordinates.	1	2	3	4	5
(14) If I have trouble on my job, I can count on my supervisor to be reasonable and give the necessary assistance.	1	2	3	4	5

Use of Resources	*Disagree*			*Agree*	
(15) Group members utilize the skills of other members.	1	2	3	4	5
(16) There is adequate time and money to meet our important goals.	1	2	3	4	5
(17) The group displays a high level of technical or professional skill required for high performance.	1	2	3	4	5
(18) Our group meetings are action-oriented and productive.	1	2	3	4	5
(19) Members are efficient in how they spend their time.	1	2	3	4	5
(20) My job makes good use of my skills and my abilities.	1	2	3	4	5
(21) People who get ahead in my department deserve to do so because of their high performance.	1	2	3	4	5
(22) When needed, we receive training in a timely manner.	1	2	3	4	5

Responsibility	*Disagree*			*Agree*	
(23) Members of my group will go out of their way to help other members achieve their goals.	1	2	3	4	5
(24) Members of my group know each other's assignments and responsibilities.	1	2	3	4	5
(25) Members of my group follow through on assignments.	1	2	3	4	5
(26) My job gives me the chance to learn new skills and techniques.	1	2	3	4	5
(27) My job allows me to identify and solve problems on my own.	1	2	3	4	5
(28) Through discussion with management, I can influence the decisions that affect my job.	1	2	3	4	5
(29) My group accepts the consequences when we make the wrong decision.	1	2	3	4	5
(30) My group actively looks for better ways to get the job done.	1	2	3	4	5
(31) I have a personal sense of responsibility to help my hospital be profitable.	1	2	3	4	5

Motivation/Pride	*Disagree*			*Agree*	
(32) We have a record of success in our group that provides a sense of pride.	1	2	3	4	5
(33) There is general group satisfaction about our contribution to the survival and future success of our hospital.	1	2	3	4	5
(34) Employee benefits are very good.	1	2	3	4	5
(35) My department recognizes those who consistently show high performance.	1	2	3	4	5
(36) I am making satisfactory progress toward my career goals.	1	2	3	4	5
(37) What happens to my hospital is important to me.	1	2	3	4	5
(38) I take personal pride in doing my job well.	1	2	3	4	5

Communications	*Disagree*			*Agree*	
(39) My group enjoys an open, honest, and direct style of communication.	1	2	3	4	5
(40) Disagreements are handled constructively, and we learn from the discussion.	1	2	3	4	5
(41) Members of my group effectively obtain, through a variety of sources, sufficient information to carry out their responsibilities.	1	2	3	4	5
(42) People at the top keep me advised of proposed solutions to problems existing at my level.	1	2	3	4	5
(43) My supervisor is aware of problems existing at my level.	1	2	3	4	5
(44) Management gives credit and recognition to people who do a good job.	1	2	3	4	5
(45) I clearly understand the employee benefits available to me.	1	2	3	4	5

Climate	*Disagree*			*Agree*	
(46) Members of my group have a high degree of respect for the competence and ability of the other members.	1	2	3	4	5
(47) My immediate supervisor treats everyone fairly.	1	2	3	4	5
(48) I can honestly disagree with management without fear of reprisal.	1	2	3	4	5
(49) Members of my work group trust each other.	1	2	3	4	5
(50) I feel that management will fairly represent my interests on issues concerned with pay and working conditions.	1	2	3	4	5

TOTAL SCORING: 225-250 Superior, 175-224 Excellent, 125-174 Average, 75-124 Fair, 0-74 Poor.

SUMMARY

In examining the various aspects of small group behavior that tend to make groups effective or ineffective, the following comparisons can be made:

Effective groups tend to have a high degree of permissiveness. This climate of permissiveness gives members an opportunity to speak their minds; they are inhibited only by normal restraints of tact, propriety, and common sense. Members of ineffective groups exhibit the opposite behavior and act restrained during meetings. They leave the meeting muttering to themselves about the ideas they did not feel free to express. The effective group assigns tasks on the basis of people's skills and interests. The ineffective group assigns tasks with little thought or planning. Effective groups exhibit intergroup status where all members share in the recognition and rewards of group achievement. To become effective, groups need successes and from successes the group builds confidence and is able to meet new challenges.[16]

CHECKLIST FOR SUPERVISORS

The following questions will require you to take a look at yourself as a supervisor. Though some of the questions are difficult, your honest answers will not only give you a good picture of your supervisory style but will also reflect the efficiency of your work group.

1. Do you have a thorough understanding of the institution's goals and your part in meeting the objectives of the institution and the budget goals for your department? Do you have full confidence in their attainment?
2. Do you avoid confusion with a clear understanding of what is expected and how to do it?
3. Do you offer suggestions or constructive criticism to your immediate supervisor and ask for additional information when necessary?
4. Do you build a team spirit and team pride by getting everyone into the act of setting goals and pulling together?
5. Are you always submerged in operational emergencies, or do you schedule times for meetings with your subordinates and your superiors?

6. Do you encourage each of your employees to come up with suggestions about ways to improve things?
7. Do you make it easy for your people to approach you with job or personal problems?
8. Do you keep your employees informed as to how they are doing?
9. Are you too busy with operational problems to be concerned with your employees' personal difficulties?
10. Do you give your employees a feeling of accomplishment by telling them how well they are doing in comparison with yesterday, or last week, or a month or year ago?
11. Do you build individual employee confidence and praise good performance, or are you afraid of being accused of sentimentality, coddling, and softsoaping?
12. Do you use personnel records and close observation to learn exactly which skills each employee has so that that employee's best abilities may be used?
13. Do you let your people know how jobs are analyzed and evaluated and what the job rates and progressions are? Do you attempt to rotate people on different jobs to build up skills for individual flexibility within the group?
14. Do you train your people for better jobs?
15. Are you developing an understudy for your job?
16. Do you hold a good person down in one position because that person may be indispensable there?
17. Do you take a chance on your people by letting them learn through mistakes, by showing a calm reaction and constructive approach to occasional failure, by encouraging them to stick their necks out without fear of the ax, and by instilling an atmosphere of confidence?
18. Do you use every opportunity to build up in your employees a sense of importance in their work?
19. Do you delegate responsibility to subordinates, or do you insist on keeping your hand in the details?
20. Do you place real responsibility on your subordinates and then hold them accountable?
21. Do you interfere with the jobs of subordinates, or do you allow them to exercise discretion and judgment in making decisions?
22. Are you doing things to discourage your subordinates?
23. Are you aware of sources of discontentment, discouragement, or frustration affecting your employees?
24. Do you listen to the ideas and reactions of subordinates with courtesy? If an idea is adopted or accepted, do you explain why?

25. Do you usually praise in public, but criticize or reprove in private? Is criticism constructive?
26. Are you aware that a feeling of belonging builds self confidence and makes people want to work harder than ever?
27. Do you ever say or do anything that detracts from the sense of personal dignity that each of your people has?

Note: The authors wish to note with thanks the contribution of Dr. Leslie M. Slote, Hartsdale, New York, in the development of a checklist similar to the one presented above.

GROUP EFFECTIVENESS REVIEW PUZZLE

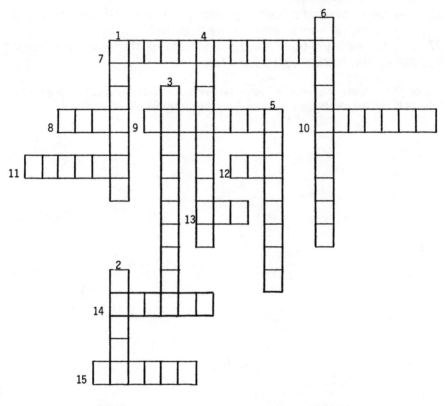

DOWN

1) A solidified communication pattern that may be called the communicative _____ order.
2) Groups need not always _____.
3) Effective meetings require this.
4) To assume you have all the right answers.
5) Watch out for communication _____.
6) To express lack of concern for a fellow group member.

ACROSS

7) What decision making should be.
8) Meetings are normally _____ oriented.
9) Takes a lot of time.
10) A group member who talks about everything but the subject.
11) A type of agenda that hinders group productivity.
12) The average executive spends _____ out of five working days in meetings.
13) Average number of hours spent in meetings per week.
14) A group member who is always complaining.
15) You are in the _____ business.

(Answers are on page 153.)

NOTES

1. Harold P. Zelko and Frank E. X. Dance, *Business and Professional Speech Communication* (New York: Holt, Rhinehart, and Winston, 1965), p. 161.

2. R. Tilman, Jr., "Problems in Review: Committees on Trial," *Harvard Business Review* 47 (1960): 162-172.

3. M. Kriesberg, "Executives Evaluate Administrative Conferences," *Advanced Management* 15 (1950): 15-17.

4. Stewart Tubbs, *A System Approach to Small Group Interaction* (Reading, Mass.: Addison-Wesley Publishing Co., 1978), p. 5.

5. Ibid.

6. Jack Gibb, "Defensive Communication," *Journal of Communication* 11 (1961): 141-148.

7. James N. Holm, *Productive Speaking for Business and the Professions* (Boston: Allyn and Bacon, Inc., 1967), p. 34.

8. Richard C. Huseman, James M. Lahiff, and John D. Hatfield, *Interpersonal Communication in Organizations* (Boston: Holbrook Press, Inc., 1976), p. 140.

9. Lester R. Bittel, "Brainstorming," *Factory Management and Maintenance* 114: 107.

10. Franklin S. Haiman, *Group Leadership and Democratic Action* (Boston: Houghton-Mifflin and Co., 1951), pp. 145-146.

11. Carl Heyel, *Encyclopedia of Management* (New York: Van Nostrand-Reinhold Co., 1971).

12. Howard H. Martin, "Communication Setting," *Speech Communication*, eds. Howard Martin and Kenneth Anderson (Boston: Allyn and Bacon, 1968), pp. 70-71.

13. Paul E. Torrence, "Function of Expressed Disagreement in Small Group Processes," *Social Forces* 35 (1957): 314-318.

14. Richard Wilhelm and Carry F. Baynes, *The I Ching* (Princeton, N.J.: Princeton University Press, 1967), p. 575.

15. Bobby R. Patton and Kim Giffin, *Problem Solving Group Interaction* (New York: Harper & Row Publishers, 1973), p. 259.

16. R. Victor Harnack and Thorrel B. Fest, *Group Discussion Theory and Technique* (New York: Appleton-Century-Crofts, 1964), pp. 177-181.

SUGGESTED READINGS

Bales, Robert F. "In Conference." *Harvard Business Review* 32: 44-50.

Bennett, James C. "The Communication Needs of Business Executives." *Journal of Business Communication* 8: 5-11.

Burke, Ronald J. "Methods of Resolving Superior-Subordinate Conflict: The Constructive Use of Subordinate Differences and Disagreements." *Organizational Behavior and Human Performance* 5: 393-411.

D'Aprix, Roger. *Employee Communication Meetings—A Handbook.* Stamford, Conn.: Xerox Corporation, 1970.

Filley, A.C. "Committee Management: Guideline from Social Science Research." *California Management Review* (Fall 1970), pp. 13-21.

Hayes, Donald, and Meltzer, Leo. "Interpersonal Judgments Based on Talkativeness: Fact or Artifact?" *Sociometry* 35: 538-561.

Kelly, J. "Make Conflict Work for You." *Harvard Business Review* 48: 103-114.

Kriesberg, Martin. "Executives Evaluate Administrative Conferences." *Advanced Management* 15: 15-17.

Loban, Lawrence N. "Questions: The Answer to Meeting Participation." *Supervision* (January 1972), pp. 11-13.

Maier, Norman. *Problem Solving Discussions and Conferences: Leadership Methods and Skills.* New York: McGraw-Hill Book Co., 1963.

Snell, Frank. *How to Hold a Better Meeting.* New York: Harper & Row, 1958.

Tillman, Rollie. "Problems in Review: Committees on Trial." *Harvard Business Review* 38: 168.

Zelko, Harold P. *Successful Conference and Discussion Techniques.* New York: McGraw-Hill Book Co., 1957.

GROUP EFFECTIVENESS REVIEW PUZZLE

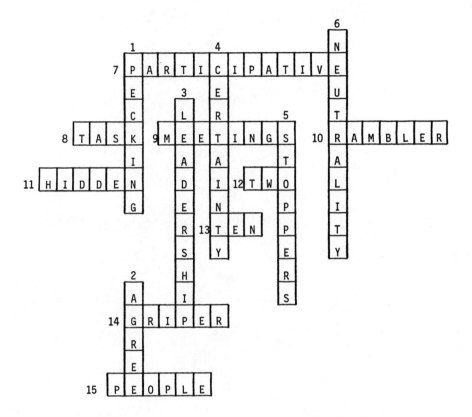

DOWN

1) A solidified communication pattern that may be called the communicative _____ order.
2) Groups need not always _____.
3) Effective meetings require this.
4) To assume you have all the right answers.
5) Watch out for communication _____.
6) To express lack of concern for a fellow group member.

ACROSS

7) What decision making should be.
8) Meetings are normally _____ oriented.
9) Takes a lot of time.
10) A group member who talks about everything but the subject.
11) A type of agenda that hinders group productivity.
12) The average executive spends _____ out of five working days in meetings.
13) Average number of hours spent in meetings per week.
14) A group member who is always complaining.
15) You are in the _____ business.

Chapter 9

Barriers to Supervisory Effectiveness

CHAPTER OBJECTIVES

The purpose of this chapter is to enable you to CHANGE your communicative behavior in a *positive* direction. After studying the material you should be able to:

Construct clearer messages.

Heighten your ability to diagnose and prescribe proper treatment for communicative illness.

Avoid communication breakdowns due to semantic differences.

Note the differences between signs and symbols.

Gain an awareness of the important differences between the verbal and situational context of messages.

Eliminate message distortion.

INTRODUCTION

The following is not a finished piece of writing. Rather it is a series of notes that were found after the death of Dr. Irving Lee of Northwestern University. They appear to be the beginning of something he was one day going to write.

Viable—capable of living or developing, as viable seeds, physically and psychologically fitted to live and grow.

I know some viable men.

They keep pushing beyond the horizons of what they already know.

They refuse to be stuck in yesterday. They won't even remain rooted in today.

They are teachable.

They keep learning. They continue to see and listen. All their horizons are temporary.

They don't deny today's wisdom—rather, they add dimensions to it.

They have strong beliefs, faith, aspirations, but they know the difference between belief and bigotry—between knowledge and dogmatism.

They are acutely aware of the limits of what they know.

They are more likely to wonder and inquire than to dismiss and deny.

They know a great deal, but they also know that they do not know it all.

I also know some stunted, deadened men.

Their outlooks have been blighted—their interest diminished—their enthusiasm restricted—their sensitivity limited.

They are old fogies, though they may be young in years.

They strive only to stay where they are.

They see only the dimensions of what has already been explored.

They search with their eyes only for what is old and familiar.

They have frozen their views in molds.

They have narrowed the wave lengths.

They are imprisoned in the little community—the little dusty dungeons of their own minds.

They are the *conflict carriers*. [1]

At times, supervisors appear to be not only the victims of their own communicative behavior, they are also the victimizers insofar as their behavior affects others. The type of communicative behavior noted above can create internal and external conflict that may become irreparable. It is therefore essential to learn to recognize the communicative signals that might eventually lead to irreparable conflict and to correct the situation before the damage has been done.

This is, of course, easier said than done. We have a strong tendency to see what we want to see and to hear what we want to hear. We not only prepare others to see and hear in a fixed way, but, more importantly, at times we allow others to predispose us to see other people as they want us to see them. Our language, our abstractions, and our mental sets cause us to not only mislead others but, at times, to be misled by others. It takes two to miscommunicate, and at times we deceive ourselves.

TYPES OF BARRIERS

Addison Bennett attempted to substantiate the assumption that certain kinds of barriers exist in health care organizations. The hypothesis was tested in a survey of 326 hospital managers who returned the mailed questionnaire. Analysis showed that the type, size, or location (rural or urban) of the hospital did not significantly influence the nature of the comments.[2]

Bennett reported that seven barriers were listed by at least ten percent of the 326 hospital managers responding to the survey:[3]

Barrier Cited	Number of Mentions*	Percent Mentioning
(1) Poor communication	145	44%
(2) Absence of training	136	42
(3) Lack of goals	93	29
(4) Lack of coordination	76	23
(5) Time constraints and work pressures	53	16
(6) Management attitudes	52	16
(7) Medical staff attitudes	31	10

*The majority of the respondents commented on more than one barrier.

SIGNS AND SYMBOLS

A special area of study called semantics is concerned with the meaning of words, that is, with the relationship between a symbol and the thing it represents, called a referent.

We use both signs and symbols to communicate. An important distinction between the two is that signs "indicate" and symbols "represent." Patients who cough, tremble, or cry out in pain are exhibiting signs that they are in distress. Nurses and physicians are constantly looking for signs in blood pressure, color of the skin, pupils of the eye, heartbeat, and so on.

When nurses and physicians verbalize these signs, they use symbols. The use of symbols is one of the basic characteristics that separates humans from animals. Humans can use symbols to communicate but animals cannot; animals can only use signs.

Gail and Michelle Myers note that

> symbols in a way are shortcuts. Imagine what it would be like if we did not have convenient shortcuts like words to communicate with one another. If I wanted to tell you something, anything at all, about an object and did not have words to name it, I would have to point to it so you would know exactly what I had in mind. Our conversation would be limited necessarily to the objects of persons or events actually present to our senses at the moment of conversation. If we did not have words at our disposal we would be extremely limited indeed. Actually we would not be much different from the animals whose survival depends upon getting around to get food, and whose communication is limited to groans and grunts.[4]

Fortunately, this condition does not hold for humans. We have developed words that enable us to communicate symbolically with one another. Imagine the dilemma of operating room nurses if there were no words to describe a particular surgical instrument and surgeons, grunting and groaning, had to look at and point to every instrument they needed.

Don Fabun estimates that there are 600,000 words in the English language today. The number is constantly growing and new expressions are constantly being coined. The number of words an adult uses in daily conversation (aside from technical words used in a profession) is about 2,000.[5]

Sanford Berman discovered that the 500 words used the most in the English language have at least 14 thousand different definitions.[6] There are about 300 million English-speaking people in the world today, and as they go about their daily lives, each of them has different experiences. Yet, even though their experiences differ, they have the same basic store of accepted symbols to use in reporting to each other what they have experienced. Each symbol must, therefore, be used to cover a wide range of meanings.[7]

Is it any wonder that at times we have communication breakdowns, conflict, misunderstanding, and deception. No two employees are alike, no two employees have the same training, no two employees have the same value system, and no two employees have the same personality or motivation. Each is unique, and it is this uniqueness that determines the personal interpretation of communicative messages. Supervisors get into trouble when they start treating employees as if they all were the same. We are not talking here about the fairness issue, but rather about one's ability to interpret and understand instructions and honestly to provide feedback to the supervisor when it is necessary.

The way we perceive determines how we communicate and the type of communication that takes place between us. Our past experiences determine which words have the most influence in the communicative message and what they mean to us. But sometimes we misinterpret because we *assume* that the person we are talking to is just like us; if something has this meaning for me, it must have the same meaning to the other person.

PEOPLE MEANING

How many times have we heard someone say, "I don't remember exactly what I said, but I know what I meant." Poor communication is the result of misinterpretation, which leads to misunderstanding. When we believe that words have meaning, we are in serious trouble. If you believe that words have meaning, try to interpret the following italicized words: "I was riding down the highway *bareback* when I was stopped by a *big hat* who thought I was a *big rigger*, but I was really a *maniac* who used to work on *bumble bees*."

If words have meaning, this statement should have meaning for you. But, for communication to be classified as effective, there must be a common code of meaning between the sender and the receiver of the message. Thus, as shown in the above statement, words do not mean, people mean; the meaning is in the person.

The statement we have cited came from the Truck Drivers Dictionary. Riding down the highway *bareback* means riding in the truck without the trailer behind it. To be stopped by a *big hat* means to be stopped by a state trooper. A *big rigger* is an arrogant truck driver. A *maniac* is a shop mechanic, and to work on *bumble bees* means to work on one-cycle engines.

Our past experiences determine which words have the most influence in the communicative message and what those words mean *to us*. When we say, "It must mean this to both of us," we may be making a faulty assumption. This is not to suggest that each and every message must be clinically analyzed. Some messages are less important than others.

Consider the following:

> I remember one day I was on my way to lunch with Dr. Petrie and as we were about to leave, Dr. Cowperthwaite stuck his head in the door to our office and said, "Hi Chuck, how are you?" Chuck Petrie stopped, thought a minute and said, "That's a very interesting and profound question. I will have to look at it from three points of view. One, how am I physically; two, how am I mentally; and three, how am I spiritually?" Cowperthwaite replied, "Chuck, I'm sorry I asked."

However, when a message is important, it should be examined for common meaning. Stuart Chase makes this point quite clear:

> A Japanese word *mokusatsu*, may have changed all our lives. It has two meanings: (1) to ignore, (2) to refrain from comment. The release of a press statement using the second meaning, in July, 1945, might have ended the war then. The emperor was ready to end it, and had the power to do so. The cabinet was prepared to accede to the Potsdam ultimatum of the Allies—surrender or be crushed—but wanted a little more time to discuss the terms. A press release was prepared announcing a policy of *mokusatsu*, with the no comment implication. But it got on the foreign wires with the *ignore* implication through a mix-up in translation: "The cabinet ignores the demand to surrender." To recall the release would have entailed the unthinkable loss of face. Had the intended meaning been publicized, the cabinet might have backed up the Em-

peror's decision to surrender. In which event, there might have been no atomic bombs over Hiroshima and Nagasaki, no Russian armies in Manchuria, no Korean War to follow. The lives of tens of thousands of Japanese and American boys might have been saved. One word, misinterpreted.[8]

THE FALLACY OF MEANING

Many times we miscommunicate because we mistakenly think the word we are using has one universal meaning, that it will mean the same to someone else as it does to us. At times, we also fail to recognize the importance of message context. We attempt to interpret words based upon the context in which they are used. The following instances underscore the importance of message context:

- This afternoon there will be a meeting in the north and south ends of the church. Children will be baptized at both ends.

- On Sunday, a special collection will be taken to defray the expenses of the new carpet. All those wishing to do something on the new carpet, come forward and get a piece of paper.

- The ladies have cast off clothing of every kind, and they may be seen in the church basement on Friday afternoon.

A story from Lewis Carroll's *Alice's Adventures in Wonderland* illustrates the importance of "people meaning:"

> "I don't know what you mean by 'glory'," Alice said. Humpty Dumpty smiled contemptuously. "Of course you don't till I tell you. I mean there is a nice knockdown argument for you." "But glory does not mean a nice knockdown argument," Alice objected. "When I use a word," Humpty Dumpty said in a rather scornful tone, "it means just what I choose it to mean—neither more nor less." "The question is," said Alice, "whether you can make words mean so many different things." "The question is," said Humpty Dumpty, "who is to be master, that's all."[9]

In this case, Humpty Dumpty was assuming, in his arrogant way, that the meaning the word held for him and the context in which it was said would be the same for Alice. He was also strongly suggesting that the word had better mean the same to Alice or she would have to answer to him. This is the type of attitude and belief that hinders the sharing of ideas and the transfer of information.

Perhaps the mistaken belief that words have meaning stems from what Irving Lee calls the "container myth:"

> If you think of words as vessels, then you are likely to talk about the meaning of a word as if the meaning were "in" that word. Assuming this, it is easy to endow words with characteristics. Just as you might say that one vessel is costlier or more symmetrical than another, you may say that one word is intrinsically more suitable for one purpose than another, or that, in and of itself, a word will have this or that meaning rather than any other. When one takes this view, he seems to say that meaning is to a word as contents are to a container.[10]

Obviously words do not contain meaning. Rather, the meaning is in the person; words in differing contexts hold different meanings for the users of those words. For instance:

- Dog: A canine animal.
- Dog: To loaf on the job.
- Dog: A clamp used on a lathe.
- Dog: To follow closely.
- Dog: A kind of sandwich.
- Dog: An andiron used in a fireplace.

MESSAGE CONTEXT

A supervisor must be able to differentiate between the "verbal" and "situational" contexts of messages. An employee tells the supervisor that a particular problem is occurring within the work group. At this same moment, the supervisor is receiving the verbal context of what is happening in the department. Now, when the supervisor directly observes what is actually taking place, senses and examines personally the existing conditions, the supervisor is receiving the situational context.

Many times after direct observation we find that the situation is much different from the one that was verbalized. This is not to say that messages should not be verbalized or passed from one source to another. But when a situation is one of utmost importance, it should be recognized that the actual conditions of the situation may not be the way they have been verbalized.

Our communication problems are compounded when we both have the same understanding of the symbol but different referents. Note in the following story how both the doctor and the patient understand the term *stomach*, yet talk past one another because of differing referents:

> "Have you ever had an operation on your stomach before?" the doctor at Memorial Hospital asked the patient. "No sir," the patient replied. Still just to be sure the doctor decided to take a few x-rays of the patient's stomach. The x-rays disclosed that the patient had only about half of his stomach left. "I thought you said that you had never had an operation on your stomach before," the doctor said firmly. "I didn't," the patient replied, "I was on my back."

Too many times we use symbols in an indiscriminate manner. Note the difficulty in answering the following questions when the referent is obscured:

- The doctor was middle-aged. How old was the doctor?
- The health care supervisor had an average income. What was the supervisor's income?
- The supervisors had a few drinks. How many did they have?
- It was a typical hospital. What was it like?
- The supervisor was average height. How tall is that?

For example, if we said we have a dog (symbol), we would both be able to envision a hairy, four-legged animal that barks. But you may be thinking of a toy poodle while we are referring to a St. Bernard (referent). Too often, we proceed on the basis of the symbols we use and develop common meaning, but, due to differing referents, we still miscommunicate. The symbols we use lack the specificity needed for precise communication.

The following story, told by Jean Vandermade at the eighth annual Hospital Topics Management Conference in Honolulu, illustrates the need for specificity in our communicative messages: A man walked into a doctor's office and the receptionist asked him what he had. He said, "Shingles." So she took his medical history, height, and weight and told him to wait. A half-hour later a nurse came in and asked him what he had. He said, "Shingles." So she took his blood pressure, gave him a blood test and an electrocardiogram, and told him to take off his clothes and wait for the doctor. A half-hour later the doctor came in and asked what he had. He said, "Shingles." The doctor asked, "Where?" He said, "Outside in the truck; where do you want them?"[11]

TECHNICAL USE OF WORDS

As we have noted, the use of symbols may be thought of as communication shortcuts, yet at times the symbols we use lack the specificity that is necessary for precise understanding. In certain vocations, this problem was resolved by developing technical language to facilitate quick and easy interpretation of messages between employees. However, here as in many other areas, people often went from one extreme to the other. That is, though symbols that are used in normal conversation may lack specificity, the use of technical language can be, and often is, too complex. This high degree of specificity is not necessary and hinders common understanding.

Have you ever wondered why a doctor says "neoplasm" instead of "cancer" or "myocardial infarction" instead of "heart attack?" According to Saul Radovsky, a suburban Boston doctor, the lingo helps to preserve the mystery of medicine. He notes that "sometimes doctors use words so obscure that even other medical people cannot understand them."[12]

Radovsky, in outlining his theory of why doctors write so poorly, gave the example of two researchers who wrote about a test they performed while attempting to learn why a boy's blood was infected:

> We used chemiluminescence assay to examine the patient's polymorphonuclear leukocyte responses to numerous particulate and soluble stimuli. The patient's polymorphonuclear leukocytes had substantially depressed chemiluminescent responses during phagocytosis of opsonized particles.[13]

The researchers were explaining that the patient's white blood cells were not generating the usual amount of light when they attacked foreign invaders in the blood stream.

There is obviously a need for technical language, but at times such a language can be too technical and too complex. Rather than facilitate a common understanding, it obscures the real meaning of the message. Many users of technical language assume that the receivers of their messages have the same understanding of the technical terms being used that they do. The following stories exemplify misunderstandings caused by the overuse of technical language.

The X-ray

Dr. Walter C. Alvarez of Mayo Clinic shares the following story:

> I remember a worrisome man who, one day, came back from the X-ray room wringing his hands and trembling with fear. "It's all up with me," he said, "the X-ray man said I have a hopeless cancer of the stomach." Knowing the roentgenologist would never have said such a thing, I asked, "Just what did he say?" and the answer was, upon dismissing him, the roentgenologist said to an assistant, "N.P." In Mayo Clinic cypher, this meant "no plates," and indicated that the X-ray man was so satisfied with the normal appearance of the stomach on the X-ray screen that he did not see any use in making films. But to the patient, watching in an agony of fear for some portent of disaster, it meant "nothing possible," in other words, the situation was hopeless.[14]

Cleaning Pipes

A plumber wrote to a government agency, "I find that hydrochloric acid quickly opens pipes. Is this a good thing to use?" A scientist at the agency replied, "The efficacy of hydrochloric acid is indubitable, but the corrosive residue is incompatible with metallic permanence."

The plumber wrote back, thanking him for the assurance that hydrochloric acid was all right. Disturbed by this turn of events, the scientist showed the letter to his boss, another scientist, who then wrote to the plumber himself, "We cannot assume responsibility for the production of toxic and noxious residue with hydrochloric acid and suggest you use an alternative procedure."

The plumber wrote back that he agreed, the hydrochloric acid worked fine. Now greatly disturbed by these misunderstandings, the scientists took the problem to their top boss. He broke the jargon and wrote to the plumber, "Don't use hydrochloric acid; it eats the hell out of pipes!"

The Thrill of Mitral Stenosis

Fred Loomis, in his book *Consultation Room,* shows the effect of technical language when communicating with a patient who is unfamiliar with the technical term being used:

> I learned something of the intricacies of plain English at an early stage of my career. A woman of 35 came in one day to tell me that she wanted a baby but that she had been told that she had a certain type of heart disease which might not interfere with a normal life but would be dangerous if she ever had a baby. From her description I thought at once of mitral stenosis. This condition is characterized by a rather distinctive rumbling murmur near the apex of the heart, and especially by a peculiar vibration felt by the examining finger on the patient's chest. The vibration is known as the "thrill" of mitral stenosis.
>
> When this woman had been undressed and was lying on my table in her white kimono, my stethoscope quickly found the heart sounds I had expected. Dictating to my nurse, I described them carefully. I put my stethoscope aside and felt intently for the typical vibration which may be found in a small but variable area of the left chest.
>
> I closed my eyes for better concentration, and felt long and carefully for the tremor. I did not find it and with my hand still on the woman's left breast, lifting it upward and out of the way, I finally turned to the nurse and said: "No thrill."
>
> The patient's black eyes snapped open, and with venom in her voice she said: "Well, isn't that just too bad? Perhaps it's just as well you don't get one. That isn't what I came for."
>
> My nurse almost choked, and my explanation still seems a nightmare of futile words.[15]

Thus, a technical language may at times be either inappropriate or overused, or both. Technical language enables two people to communicate quickly and concisely, but only to the extent that both parties have the same communicative code. When they have the same code, they have common understanding, and their messages are being transferred and interpreted as they were intended to be transferred and interpreted. Remember that words have more than a single use; one word can mean many different things. Language is constantly changing, and new words are constantly being coined. An anonymous poet perhaps said it best in the following lines:

Remember when hippie meant big in the hips,
And a trip involved travel in cars, planes, and ships?
When pot was a vessel for cooking things in,
And hooked was what grandmother's rugs may have been?
When fix was a verb that meant mend or repair,
And be-in meant merely existing somewhere?
When neat meant well organized, tidy and clean,
And grass was ground cover, normally green?
When groovy meant furrowed with channels and hollows?
And birds were winged creatures, like robins and swallows?
When fuzz was a substance, real fluffy, like lint,
And bread came from bakeries and not from the mint?
When roll meant a bun, and rock was a stone,
And hang-up was something you did with the phone?
It's groovy man, groovy, but English it's not.
Methinks our language is going to pot.

THE PROCESS OF ABSTRACTION

As communicators, we are constantly abstracting information selectively. We select specific bits and pieces of information based on our feelings, needs, and attitudes. Thus, we predispose ourselves to see things in a specific way. At other times, we allow others to predispose us in the way they wish to be seen, to persuade us to see them as they want us to see. In this way, we develop mental sets (we can see something in only one way) and are misled. We allow ourselves to be deceived. Richard C. Huseman, James H. Lahiff, and John D. Hatfield explain this deceptive selection process in this way:

The fact that we perceive selectively limits the quantity of stimuli to which we will attach meaning. That such selectivity is necessary is obvious when one considers the thousands of stimuli one is exposed to each day. Since it is not humanly possible to attach meaning to them all, it becomes the receiver's task to select those stimuli to attend. This determination and selection are made on the basis of which ones are most meaningful to the receiver.[16]

Thus, we see and hear what we want to hear; we select. We see and hear what we are prepared to see and hear. Again, we select—no one else. Consider the following triangles:

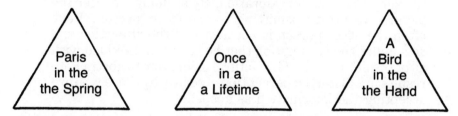

Our familiarity with the statements in each of the three triangles predisposes us to read them in a fixed way. Reread them. Do you notice anything unusual? If you noticed the extra word in each triangle, you are more observant than most. Most people who read the triangles miss the extra word because they are predisposed to see the statements as they normally see them. This kind of mental set also occurs in our communication with others. Thus, we should learn to become more aware of our development of these sets.

How accurately you receive messages is determined by your abstractions. You are constantly abstracting, and these abstractions may develop into mental sets that limit your ability to see the truth. Consider the following:

- F-O-L-K spells _____.
- P-O-L-K spells _____.
- The white of an egg is called the _____.

The white of an egg is called the *albumen*. However, most people respond by saying *yolk*. Again, they are predisposed to see something in a fixed way, and therefore they saw it that way. Try two more. The answers will be given at the end of the chapter:

- Try to make *one* word out of the two words, new door.

- Name *only two* U.S. coins that total 55 cents; one of them is not a nickel.

Huseman, Lahiff, and Hatfield contend that

> an effective communicator is one who remains aware that he is abstracting. While it should be obvious that this process is necessary, we should also recognize the high cost that accompanies it. The cost of abstracting is that we sacrifice many details, some of which may be relevant to the subject under consideration. By so doing we alter the picture we are transmitting to the other person. Very often the other person is not aware of the alteration and acts under the assumption that he has been provided with all of the details. . . . This natural inclination to abstraction results in a distorted perception of reality by those who are accepting the information as gospel.[17]

Why do we develop these mental sets so easily? We have already noted that it is necessary to abstract, that our abstractions are based on our biases, our value systems, our beliefs, and our attitudes. The following story may indicate an additional reason for allowing ourselves to become predisposed through abstractions. This famous story about Mulla Nasrudin opens with a man looking at Nasrudin searching on the ground:

> "What have you lost, Mulla?" the man asked.
> "My key," said the Mulla.
> So they both went down on their knees and looked for it. After a time the man asked, "Where exactly did you drop it?"
> "In my house."
> "Then why are you looking here?"
> "There is more light here than inside my own house."[18]

At times we develop mental sets that we know are not accurate, but we keep them because they are comfortable. We know we are not seeing the truth, but we subconsciously push truth to the back of our mind. We quickly latch on to what we want to see because there's more light there and it's easier and less painful to see. If we were to look where truth lies, it would take much more effort to analyze, decipher, and accept. We might have to go deeper into our value system than we want to. Of course, we all know that sooner or later the real problem must be dealt with, but for now it's much easier to look where there is more light—the light allows us to see what we want to see even though we know we are looking in the wrong place.

You may recall that in Chapter 7 we discussed the communication flow between supervisors and employees. The conclusions of two studies mentioned in that chapter are worth recalling here.

Anthony Downs, in his Rand Corporation monograph, states that communication distortion takes place not only in a downward pattern but in an upward pattern as well. Subordinates will facilitate upward-directed messages that they believe will either please the boss or enhance their own welfare. On the other hand, superiors will suppress messages directed to subordinates if they perceive such messages as having a deleterious effect upon themselves or the organization.[19] This conclusion was supported by P. Krivonos, who surveyed the findings of upward-communication research and concluded:

- Subordinates tend to distort information upward in a manner that pleases their superiors.

- Subordinates tend to tell their superiors what they want them to know.

- Subordinates tend to tell their superiors what they think they want to hear.

- Subordinates tend to tell their superiors information that reflects favorably on themselves and/or does not reflect negatively on themselves.[20]

This is not meant to suggest that all employees are dishonest and untruthful. On the contrary, most are direct, honest, and can be trusted to provide accurate feedback when it is requested. Yet at times supervisors still receive distorted information. This is a result of the abstraction process, by which supervisors are predisposed by others to see what they want the supervisors to see. Supervisors need to develop an awareness of this phenomenon in order to deal with it.

SUGGESTED REMEDIES

We can eliminate much of the distortions in our communications if we remember these reciprocal points:

> Words, in and of themselves, have no meaning.
> People should not be word-minded.
> People should be person-minded.
> Meaning is in the person.

Supervisors should never ask subordinates if they understand. When they do so, the pressure is on the subordinates to respond affirmatively; the question calls for a predisposed answer. If the subordinates respond negatively, they may feel that their supervisors will think that they are ignorant. If they respond positively, their supervisors will think they understand when in fact they may not.

Rather than, "Do you understand?" ask, "What do you understand?" This forces the receiver of the message to repeat the message to the satisfaction of the sender, thereby ensuring a common understanding.

Always remember to

- recognize the difference between the verbal and situational context of messages,

- question and paraphrase important messages,

- seek feedback, and

- realize that you are abstracting by placing more emphasis on some words than others (your receiver may not be abstracting in the same manner).

It might be said that at times we think too much. Over the years, we have learned to become extremely analytical, and we tend to suggest all kinds of logical answers for an employee's unusual behavior. In this process of developing our thinking patterns, we often neglect our sensing side, which can be a valuable tool for every health care supervisor. Consider the following story.

The anthropologist Castaneda complains to his teacher, Don Juan.

"For years I have truly tried to live in accordance with your teachings. Obviously I have not done well. How can I do better now?"

"You think and talk too much. You must stop talking to yourself."

"What do you mean?"

"You talk to yourself too much. You're not unique at that. Everyone of us does that. We carry on an internal talk. Think about it. Whenever you are alone, what do you do?"

"I talk to myself."

"What do you talk to yourself about?"

"I don't know; anything, I suppose."

"I'll tell you what we talk to ourselves about. We talk about our world. In fact we maintain our world with our internal talk."

"How do we do that?"

"Whenever we finish talking to ourselves the world is always as it should be. We renew it, we kindle it with life, we uphold it with internal talk. Not only that, but we also choose our paths as we talk to ourselves. Thus we repeat the same choices over and over until the day we die, because we keep on repeating the same internal talk over and over until the day we die."

"A warrior is aware of this and strives to stop his talking. This is the last point you have to know if you want to live like a warrior."

"How can I stop talking to myself?"

"First of all you must use your ears to take some of the burden from your eyes. We have been using our eyes to judge the world since the time we were born. We talk to others and to ourselves mainly about what we see. A warrior is aware of that and listens to the world; he listens to the sounds of the world."[21]

This story suggests that at times we structure, we develop mental sets that destroy our ability to be flexible, to see things from a different perspective. We put everything into a specific category or box. Through our internal talk (thinking), we structure our world as we want it to be. In some situations, this is appropriate behavior. However, certain situations or conditions may arise that require little thinking and much sensing. In such situations, it is the sensing side that will enable you to break your mental set, recognize your tunnel vision, and solve a problem with a fresh approach. Fritz Perls has noted that "ultimate awareness can only take place if the computer is gone, if the intuition, the awareness is so bright that one really comes to his senses. The empty mind in Eastern philosophy is worthy of highest praise. So lose your mind and come to your senses."[22]

We are not suggesting that supervisors stop thinking. Rather, supervisors should work hard to develop a balance between thinking and sensing (feeling). Their communicative behaviors should be determined by the situation. In some situations, it is best to think in a structured, logical way. But, in other situations, thinking will not help you much if there appears to be no answers for the particular problem, no computer print-out sheets to provide you with data, no experts to provide advice. In these situations, you have to "come to your senses." Listen to the situational variables that are around you and then reflect, but not in the old stereotyped fashion that you are used to. Look for new information, You have to have good "sense" to solve some problems.

AN IMPORTANT DISTINCTION

As we move toward the end of the twentieth century, communication gets blamed increasingly whenever something goes wrong. A popular refrain is, "We had a communication breakdown." At times this is obviously true, but at other times apparently "good" communication indeed turns out to be "poor" communication.

The key to this perceptual dilemma lies in the word *meaning*. The goal of every communicative act is the transfer of a common meaning between the sender and receiver of the message. However, at times we may be reprimanded or offered constructive criticism that we do not fully appreciate. It is at such moments that we are likely to say, "We had a communication breakdown," when, in fact, there was no breakdown at all. The common meaning was there, the communicative act was clear, but our displeasure evoked a response of poor communication when the communication could not have been clearer.

It is thus important to be able to distinguish between good communication with a common understanding and poor communication with little or no understanding.

Earlier in this chapter you were asked to solve two puzzles:

- Try to make *one* word out of the two words, new door. Answer: One word.

- Name *only two* U.S. coins that total 55 cents; one of them is not a nickel. Answer: The one that is not a nickel is a 50-cent piece.

If you had difficulty figuring out the answers to the two puzzles, the reason is that you probably perceived each answer in a literal context rather than a figurative one. In dealing with employees, supervisors frequently decode the employees' messages literally, then find out much later that the employees were actually communicating on a figurative wave-length.

BARRIERS REVIEW PUZZLE

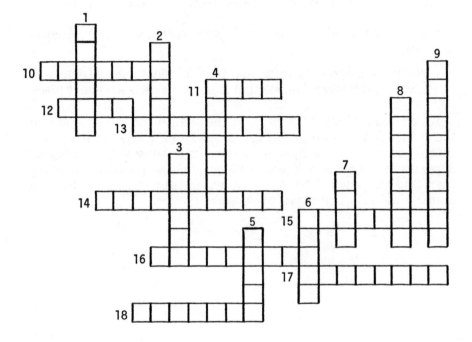

DOWN

1) Good communication always produces this type of meaning between people.
2) The employment of language.
3) Who has meaning?
4) What you should be sensitive to.
5) Indicates rather than represents.
6) Words have what type of usage?
7) Never ask, "Do you understand?" It is better to ask, "_____ do you understand?"
8) What represents a word symbol?
9) To check communication.

ACROSS

10) Words or things that stand for something not present.
11) Without this people have no meaning.
12) We miscommunicate because we think words have _____ usage.
13) The study of the meaning of words.
14) A communication barrier.
15) What communication conveys.
16) A type of word usage.
17) When communicating we should always seek to _____ meaning.
18) Do not think of words in this manner.

(Answers are on page 179.)

NOTES

1. Irving Lee, *Handling Barriers in Communication* (New York: Harper & Row, 1957), pp. 148-149.
2. Addison Bennett, "Toward More Effective Management: A Special Study in Management Problems and Practices," *Hospital Topics*, July 1973, p. 15.
3. Ibid.
4. Gail Myers and Michelle Myers, *The Dynamics of Human Communication* (New York: McGraw-Hill Book Co., 1973), p. 54.
5. Don Fabun, *Communications* (Beverly Hills, Calif.: The Glencoe Press, 1968), pp. 27-28.
6. Sanford Berman, *Understanding and Being Understood* (San Diego, Calif.: International Communication Institute, 1965), p. 14.
7. Fabun, *Communications*, p. 28.
8. Stuart Chase, *The Power of Words* (New York: Harcourt, Brace and World, Inc., 1954), pp. 4-5.
9. Lewis Carroll, *Alice's Adventures in Wonderland, Through the Looking Glass, and the Hunting of the Snark* (New York: Modern Library, Inc., 1925), pp. 246-247.
10. Irving Lee, "On a Mechanism of Misunderstanding," *Promoting Growth Toward Maturity in Interpreting What Is Read*, ed. Gray (Chicago: University of Chicago Press, 1951), pp. 86-90.
11. Jean Vandermade, "Up-date Asepsis in Patient Care: IV, Hyperalimentation and Urinary Catheter" (Paper presented at the eighth annual *Hospital Topics* Management Conference, Honolulu, 1980).
12. Saul Radovsky, "Medical Writing: Another Look," *New England Journal of Medicine* 301, no. 3, p. 134.
13. Saul Radovsky, *The News and Observer*, July 22, 1979.
14. Walter C. Alvarez, *Nervousness, Indigestion, and Pain* (New York: Harper & Row, 1954), p. 56.
15. Frederic Loomis, *Consultation Room* (New York: Alfred A. Knopf, Inc., 1939), p. 47.
16. Richard C. Huseman, James H. Lahiff, and John D. Hatfield, *Interpersonal Communication in Organizations* (Boston: Holbrook Press, Inc., 1976), p. 27.
17. Ibid., pp. 58-59.
18. Idnies Shah, *The Exploits of the Incomparable Mulla Nasrudin* (New York: E.P. Dutton, 1972), p. 26.
19. Anthony Downs, *Inside Bureaucracy* (Santa Monica, Calif.: Rand Corporation, 1964), pp. 118-123.
20. P. Krivonos, "Distortion of Subordinate to Superior Communication" (Paper presented at a meeting of the International Communication Association, Portland, Ore., 1976).
21. Carlos Castaneda, *A Separate Reality: Further Conversations with Don Juan* (New York: Simon and Schuster, 1971), pp. 262-263.
22. Joen Fagen and Irma Lee Shepard, eds., *Gestalt Therapy Now* (New York: Harper & Row, 1971), p. 38.

SUGGESTED READINGS

Berman, Sanford I. *Understanding and Being Understood*. San Diego, Calif.: International Communication Institute, 1965.

Chase, Stuart, *The Power of Words*. New York: Harcourt, Brace and World, Inc., 1954.

Fleishman, Alfred. *Sense and Nonsense: A Study in Human Communication*. San Francisco: International Society for General Semantics, 1971.

Frogman, Robert. "How to Say What You Mean; Business Communication." *Nation's Business* 45: 76-78.

_____. "Prevent Short Circuits When You Talk." *Nation's Business* 51: 88-89.

_____. "Make Words Fit the Job." *Nation's Business* 47: 76-79.

Hayakawa, S.I. *The Use and Misuse of Language*. New York: Fawcett World Library: Crest, Gold Medal, and Premier Books, 1962.

Heyel, C. "How to Communicate Better with Employees." *American Business Communication Bulletin* 37, no. 2: 38-40.

Johnson, Wendell. "The Fateful Process of Mr. A. Talking to Mr. B." *Harvard Business Review* 31: 49-56.

Laporte, Jeanne. "Participatory Management—The Technique to Alleviate Alienation of Bureaucratic Organizations." Thesis, University of Ottawa, Ontario, May 1972.

Lee, Irving J. *How to Talk With People*. New York: Harper & Row, 1952.

_____, and Lee, Laura L. *Handling Barriers in Communication*. New York: Harper & Row, 1957.

Maier, Norman R. S.; Hoffman, L. Richard; Hooven, John J.; and Read, William H. *Superior-Subordinate Communication in Management, Report No. 52*. New York: American Management Association, 1961, p. 9.

Minteer, Catherine. *Understanding in a World of Words*. San Francisco: International Society for General Semantics, 1970.

Odgen, C.K., and Richard, I.A. *The Meaning of Meaning*. New York: Harcourt, Brace and World, Inc., 1952.

Roethlisberger, Fritz J. "Barriers to Communication Between Men." *Northwestern University Information* 20, no. 25.

Rogers, Carl. "Communication: Its Blocking and Facilitation." *Northwestern University Information* 20, no. 25: 9-15.

Weaver, C.H. "Measuring Point of View as a Barrier to Communication." *Journal of Communication* 7, no. 1: 5-13.

Wiksell, Wesley. *Do They Understand You?* New York: McMillan and Co., 1960.

BARRIERS REVIEW PUZZLE

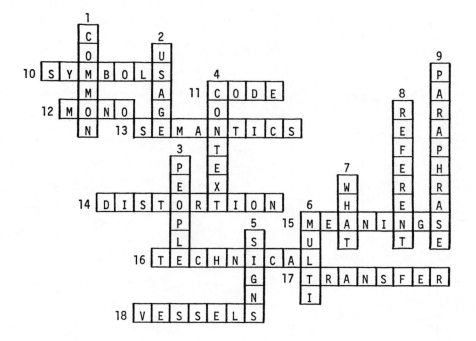

DOWN

1) Good communication always produces this type of meaning between people.
2) The employment of language.
3) Who has meaning?
4) What you should be sensitive to.
5) Indicates rather than represents.
6) Words have what type of usage?
7) Never ask, "Do you understand?" It is better to ask, "_____ do you understand?"
8) What represents a word symbol?
9) To check communication.

ACROSS

10) Words or things that stand for something not present.
11) Without this people have no meaning.
12) We miscommunicate because we think words have _____ usage.
13) The study of the meaning of words.
14) A communication barrier.
15) What communication conveys.
16) A type of word usage.
17) When communicating we should always seek to _____ meaning.
18) Do not think of words in this manner.

Chapter 10

How to Interview: The First Step to Better Placement

CHAPTER OBJECTIVES

The purpose of this chapter is to enable you to CHANGE your communicative behavior in a *positive* direction. After studying the material you should be able to:

Create a favorable interview climate.

Have a thorough understanding of the five stages of the interviewing process.

Assess the types of interviewing questions that can be used.

Nurture better job placement.

Gain more effective job interviews.

Eliminate common interviewing mistakes.

INTRODUCTION

Each new employee provides the supervisor with an opportunity to strengthen the effectiveness of the work team. Too often, one hears supervisors complain that "the personnel department does the hiring." Yet the final responsibility for hiring must lie with the potential employee's immediate supervisor. Given the importance of the employment interview, it is disturbing to note that most supervisors are not equipped to handle interviewing because of a lack of understanding of and minimal training in interviewing techniques.

THE EFFECTIVE EMPLOYMENT INTERVIEW

It will help to review some key steps to follow in the employment interview. The supervisor who wishes to be effective in the employment interview should do the following.

- Set a plan. Structure the interview to obtain maximum information and cover all necessary areas.

- Review the job specification or job description. There is nothing more fatal to positive results than to enter the employment interview with little knowledge of the job requirements. If the personnel department has not provided you with a written description of the job, then write one yourself.

- Don't begin the interview until you have reviewed the job application. Have the applicant wait outside your office while you review the application form, any tests administered by your personnel department, and any reference checks made in advance.

- Pick the right place for an interview. It should be held in private. Limit phone calls that can disturb the applicant and interrupt your train of thought. Ensure that you have enough time (30 to 45 minutes).

- Familiarize yourself with the five logical segments of the employment interview (warm-up stage, applicant-talking stage, questioning stage, employer informational stage, wind-up stage).

- Keep in mind that it is not necessary for you to impress the applicant with the importance of your position. This means you are going to have to control the amount of time you talk as compared with the amount of time that the applicant is permitted to talk.

- Watch the level of your language. Speak *to* the applicant in terms easy to understand, not above or beneath the applicant's level.

- Watch your biases; don't let them get in the way of your ability to select the best qualified applicant.

- Don't be hesitant about making notes. Make a record of essential facts and judgments during and after the interview.

Arthur R. Pell once wrote that an interview has four major purposes: (1) to get information, (2) to evaluate the applicant, (3) to give information, and (4) to make a friend.[1] In many interviews, only one or two of these purposes are satisfied while the rest remain unfulfilled.

If you are going to make an intelligent placement decision, you must obtain maximum information from the applicant. This requires sensitive listening skills. The ratio of interviewer talking to interviewer listening is critical. In the average 45-minute interview, the applicant should talk more than half the time. Since it is equally important for the applicant to judge you and your firm or institution, it is essential that the applicant receive basic information about the job, the institution, and career opportunities.

As important as eliciting and giving information is the evaluation process. It is not uncommon for the supervisor's personal bias to intrude upon the effective evaluation of a candidate. Biases can be favorable or unfavorable. We often like certain things about people and, therefore, are impressed when an applicant shows one of those favorable traits. Some of us are impressed by the way applicants dress or comb their hair. Still others are sensitive to speech mannerisms. (How often have you been impressed by someone with an English accent?)

Some interviewers rely on pseudoscience and mythology. Too many interviewers believe they can detect "the criminal type" or they harbor prejudices against fat people (they are either jovial or lethargic!) or against redheads (they are always unintelligent!). The "natural" judgments of character are as unreliable as the myths about such judgments. Quite obviously, appearance is not a reliable predictor of personality traits.

The intrusion of personal bias and pseudoscience has led to an alarming proportion of "quick sets." Very often interviewers allow their initial impression of a candidate to influence their final decision. One researcher found that most personnel interviewers made their decisions after just 4 minutes of a 15-minute interview.[2] This is unfortunate because very often an initial impression is positively or negatively affected by intensive exploration with the candidate over a much longer period. This brings to mind the silent screen star whose good looks and swashbuckling manner produced an aura of masculinity but whose soprano voice doomed his career when talking movies were introduced. The opposite is often true as well. An individual who may not look the part may very well be just the person for the job.

Some supervisors are reluctant to vary their approach to interviews. Stereotyping interviews—that is, falling into a comfortable routine—often is nonproductive because of the different types of people who present themselves for interviews. The successful interviewer is flexible in approach and tries to be aware of the applicant's personality and needs.

According to Pell, one purpose of the interview is to "make a friend."[3] Keep in mind that every unsuccessful applicant is often a member of the community served by your institution. Impressions made in the interview situation are lasting ones. Common courtesy, a dignified approach, and a sympathetic rejection will be remembered even though the job was not offered. For the applicant who is successful, first impressions of the institution—usually obtained in the initial interview—are brought into the work area and can aid in developing an efficient and dedicated employee. When you interview an applicant for employment, you are functioning as a public relations arm of the institution. Dignified interviews, with ample opportunity for the applicants to present their credentials, will be of immeasurable encouragement to the new employees in an institution.

FIVE STAGES OF THE INTERVIEW

The Warm-Up Stage

It is essential that you establish rapport with the candidate, who is often apprehensive about the interview. Diving into a cold pool can be quite a shock; it is often best to wade into cold water. It is important to remember this when applicants come in and identify themselves to you. Most applicants are tense, and tension will affect the productivity of the interview. It is essential that you invest the time to put the applicant at ease.

This can be accomplished in many ways. Make an effort to establish a proper setting for the interview. If you seem harried and give the impression that the interview is a necessary evil, then the applicant will be defensive and often unresponsive. Talk about the weather; talk about transportation—ask if the applicant found it easy to get to the institution or found your office without difficulty. Don't have the applicant sit and wait while you look over the application blank; review the form before the applicant comes into the room. Don't open the interview with a caustic or insensitive question.

When someone asks how long the warm-up period should take, the best reply is, "As long as it will take to put the applicant at ease and in a nondefensive frame of mind." Sometimes you may be able to base your warm-up question on an item that appears in the application blank. Move on to the next stage when the applicant is talking and freely exchanging information with you.

The Applicant-Talking Stage

Once again, refer to the application blank or ask an open-ended question. Questions that can be answered with a simple "yes" or "no" are not effective. Rather, say, "I see that you worked at Metropolitan General Hospital for three years. Can you tell me about your job and what you did there?"

Now is the crucial test—can you keep your mouth shut? The idea is to let the applicant talk; let the applicant set the pace. The extent to which you may have to ask questions and guide the interview will depend entirely on the applicant. There will be enormous pressure on you to keep the conversation flowing, and there will be the problem almost all inexperienced interviewers face—handling periods of silence. It is strongly advised that you resist the temptation to step into the breach. The applicant will eventually move on, and then very often will reveal critical points about his or her character or experiences.

The Questioning Stage

There is no set combination of questions that will be satisfactory for every interview. Pell gives us a most helpful review of the six types of questions applicable in most situations.

1. *The "W" questions:* "What?" "When?" "Where?" "Who?" and "Why?"—coupled with "How?"—are useful in most interviewing situations.
2. *Leading questions:* Too often these questions move applicants to give the answers that they think the interviewer wants. Leading questions should be discouraged, but they may be used to control the interview or to stop digression.
3. *Probing questions:* These are incisive and specific questions used to obtain more detail about a specific activity or area. When a probing question is asked, the interviewer should be quite familiar with the area being examined.
4. *Yes-No questions:* This type of question should be used sparingly. A yes-no question cannot stand alone, since the form of the question does not give the applicant the opportunity to expand the answer.
5. *Situational questions:* The interviewer poses hypothetical problems and encourages the applicant to answer. In so doing, the applicant reveals knowledge and understanding of a subject. This type of question can be effective if the hypothetical problem is close to reality.
6. *Clarification and reflection questions:* This type of questioning essentially "mirrors" the interviewee's answers. It is used to get a fuller understanding of a question previously answered.[4]

It is a good idea to prepare your questions in advance of the interview. It is nonproductive to overload the applicant with a series of rapid-fire questions so that the interviewee is forced to remember three or four questions posed in succession. Again, remember that the successful interviewer speaks far less than the applicant, even when giving information about the job. This often gives the applicant an opportunity to ask questions and make comments that can be evaluated.

It is most helpful in the questioning stage to give applicants the impression that you are genuinely interested in their background. This can be accomplished by putting yourself in the applicant's position. Remember the strain of an interview when you were on the other side of the table? Beware of being argumentative in this "drawing out" stage. If you disagree with an answer, it is not essential for you to correct the applicant or to argue. If you feel that the applicant is holding back information, not telling the complete truth, it may be best to avoid a confrontation and instead to assume a sympathetic posture. This can result in finally arriving at the complete and true story.

Employer Informational Stage

Supervisors often forget that there are two decisions to be made in an interview. The first is the supervisor's decision as to the match: Does the applicant fit the job? Should an offer be made? The second decision is one that falls to the applicant: Do I want to work for this institution?

It is essential that the supervisor provide the applicant with all pertinent information concerning the job itself and the institution in general. Tell the applicant the what, why, how, and when of the job and answer any questions. This can be a most revealing part of the interview, since applicants' questions often are indicative of their value systems.

Too often this part of the interview is rushed or underrated. Too many times, newly hired employees have been heard to state that the job to which they are assigned is quite different from the job explained to them in the interview.

A most helpful tool in the informational stage of the interview is a job description and, if one is available, a job specification. The job description often contains a job summary section that gives the applicant (and most important, the interviewer) an overall concept of the purpose, nature, and extent of the task to be performed. It also shows how the job differs generally from others in the organization. The job specification is also invaluable, as it contains the personal requirements, necessary skills, and the physical demands of the job. The job specification form commonly includes the requirements for education, experience, initiative, and ingenuity. Physical demands, working demands, and unavoidable hazards are outlined. A job description and a job specification are indispensable to the interview and placement process.

It is incorrect to assume that a supervisor and a subordinate are in fair agreement about the nature of the subordinate's job when they are discussing some plan or decision affecting the subordinate's work. A study conducted on superior-subordinate communications in management concluded that

> . . . if a single answer can be drawn from the detailed research study (presented in the report) into superior-

subordinate communication on the managerial level in business, it is this: If one is speaking of the subordinate's specific job—his duties, the requirements he must fulfill in order to do his job well, his intelligent anticipation of future changes in his work, and the obstacles which prevent him from doing as good a job as possible—the answer is that he and his boss do not agree or differ more than they agree in almost every area.[5]

This kind of misunderstanding too often starts at the original placement phase. Applicants should be absolutely certain about the duties and requirements of the job for which they are being interviewed; this is the responsibility of the immediate supervisor who will make the placement choice.

In either this stage or the previous one, there are questions that can be extremely helpful in revealing the applicant's lifestyle, personal philosophy, and general character. For example:

- What books have you read over the last six months?

- Looking back over the last several years, what is the most important way in which you have changed in that time?

- Where do you want to be—as far as your work is concerned—in the next three years, five years, ten years?

- What are some of the things you do when you are not working—your hobbies and outside interests?

The Wind-Up Stage

To know when and how to conclude an interview comes with experience. The inexperienced supervisor will often end an interview abruptly and many times on a less than positive note. Be careful not to abort an interview based on a very quick, surface evaluation of the applicant. It may well be that, in so doing, you will cut down the amount of time spent in the interview because it is obvious that the individual being interviewed is not up to the standards of the job. But many years of experience in interviewing at all levels has demonstrated that intuition and initial feelings are not the best guides for proper placement. Sometimes an applicant takes a long time to warm up, and initial negative vibrations change much later in the interview. It is your duty to give applicants a fair chance to reveal a *complete* picture of their qualifications, motivations, and aspirations. It is also important that you not let the interview drag on, that you close at the right time, that you end on a positive note, and that you leave the applicant with a positive impression of your institution.

THE DO'S AND DON'TS IN JOB INTERVIEWING

At this juncture, it is helpful to list those factors that make an interview successful and productive and those that are counterproductive to sound placement.

- Do not stereotype your interview.
- Do not allow the interview to assume the character of a comfortable routine.
- Do not fall back on selecting only those candidates who show previous experience similar to that required by the job in question.
- Do not overhire. That is, do not select someone whose ability far exceeds that required by the job.
- Do not be overly formal. Getting the applicant to relax is essential for a productive interview.
- Do not give advice to the applicant. This is a preemployment stage, and your only responsibility is to *select* a candidate appropriate for the position.
- Do not be impatient. Let the interview run as long as necessary to develop a proper evaluation of the candidate.
- Do maintain control over the interview. If the conversation is wandering, bring the applicant back on the track. If the applicant's responses are too general, ask for relevant details.
- Do familiarize yourself with the job specification and job qualifications.
- Do prepare in advance for the interview, permitting enough time and enough privacy.
- Do not speak more than the applicant does. A good gauge would be to limit your talking to one-third of the time (anything less than half of the time will do).

- Do leave the applicant with a favorable impression of the institution.

- Do not set inappropriate standards for the job—either too high or too low.

- Do not judge the applicant by one favorable or unfavorable attribute (the "halo" effect is detrimental to overall evaluation).

- Do know your biases and do not let them interfere with the evaluation process.

- Do not reach a conclusion before the interview has started (this happens more often than we are willing to admit) or before the interview has been completed.

- Do not reveal by word or expression that you are critical of the applicant's responses.

- Do not interrupt unless the applicant is wandering or is not specific.

- Do review, in advance of the interview, the application form and any personnel tests or references.

In any list of don'ts, it can be helpful to review some of the mistakes that inexperienced interviewers make. Arthur Witkin, an industrial psychologist, presents six classic mistakes:

1. The interviewer "telegraphs" the answer expected on each question. This results in a yes-no response.
2. The interviewer tries to scare or intimidate applicants by setting up traps. Very little will be revealed about the applicants' real selves because they will be too busy defending to reveal anything.
3. The interviewer does all the telling—about the company, about the job, about the interviewer's own work and family. Such interviewers are in love with the sound of their own voices.
4. The interviewer is so busy writing down every word the applicant utters that there is no time for listening, looking, and reacting. After the interview, the interviewer really doesn't know what kind of person the applicant is.
5. The interviewer is busy filling out an application blank. The interview consists of getting references, statistics, salaries, and dates.

6. The interviewer believes in intuition or is a "stargazer." This interviewer sees qualities in the applicant that no one else is able to see.[6]

THE SCREENING INTERVIEW

In situations where a great number of applicants apply, it is important to conduct a screening of the candidates as quickly as possible to save time for the supervisor and the applicants. In many instances, the personnel department is responsible for the preliminary screening, but there may be occasions when this is the supervisor's responsibility. Here, briefly, are the three objectives of the screening interview:

1. to determine whether the job applicant is *generally* qualified for a specific job opening
2. to determine whether the job applicant is qualified for other present or future openings in the department or in the institution
3. to make a favorable impression on the job applicant (it is essential to create a favorable public relations impact on all applicants who contact the institution for a job)

The screening interview is designed to limit the number of applicants to be given a placement interview. While recruitment is a magnet—its prime objective is to attract as many candidates as possible—screening is more like a sieve that lets through only those candidates who might well qualify for the job. It is important that applicants feel their candidacies have been reasonably considered. Therefore, although the screening interview is short, it should not be uncomfortably rushed.

One of the best ways to expedite the screening interview is to identify those elements in the candidate's qualifications most crucial in determining possible suitability for the job. For example, the nature of the position may require the employee to work overtime or to work unusual hours. If the interviewer spends 30 minutes determining the applicant's technical knowledge and experience and then finds out that the applicant is unwilling to work the required hours, valuable time has been wasted. It is important to recognize that the screening interview is merely an opportunity to determine, in a rather *general* way, whether or not the applicant is qualified for the job opening. Intensive consideration of technical qualifications and personality should be left for later stages of the interview or for the placement interview. The primary objective of the *screening* interview is to put the candidate at ease and to determine as rapidly as possible if that candidate meets the basic requirements. The purpose of the *placement* interview is to determine specifically and in depth whether the applicant's work habits, attitudes, and personality are compatible with the job and with the institution.

AFFIRMATIVE ACTION

You and the applicant are not alone in the employment interview; sitting in are unseen but still powerful participants—the federal government and its partner, the state government. Various legislative acts affect the employment interview and, more importantly, circumscribe kinds of behavior that may have been possible prior to the enactment of such legislation.

It is now firmly established, if not finally interpreted, that employers must make a special effort to hire individuals who are deemed to be in a "protected class." The law defines a protected class as one of several minorities that have been subjected to discrimination in hiring and promotion in past years: blacks, Spanish-surnamed Americans, Asian Americans, American Indians, and women. Special emphasis is placed on the several areas of the employment process where rejection is possible. These sensitive areas are

- in the general prescreening of applicants through replies to ads, walk-in candidates, or any other system of applying for a job
- in the most controversial arena of testing
- in the two forms of selection interviews—screening and placement
- in any checks—such as security checks, reference checks, or physical examinations—that may result in rejection

Affirmative action is mandated by federal, state, and local laws, as well as by presidential executive orders and court decisions. It would be most helpful if the supervisor were provided with the operative legislation in the area of equal employment opportunity, such as:

- Title VII of the Civil Rights Act of 1964, as amended by the Equal Employment Opportunity Act of 1972. Your institution is very likely covered by these acts, since they apply to organizations engaged in interstate commerce and employing 15 or more persons; all educational institutions, public and private; state and local governments; public and private employment agencies; labor unions with 15 or more members; and joint labor-management committees for apprenticeship and training.

- Executive Order 11246, as amended by Executive Order 11375. This affects federal contractors and subcontractors with 50 or more employees and contracts of $50,000 or more. The orders require an employer to have an approved affirmative action program on file with the Office of Federal Contract Compliance Programs.

- The Equal Pay Act of 1963 as amended by the Education Amendments of 1972 (Section 6(d) of the Fair Labor Standards Act). This specifically requires that organizations pay their female employees, both those exempt and nonexempt from the Fair Labor Standards Act, the same salary that their male employees receive for doing basically similar work.

- The Age Discrimination and Employment Act of 1967, as amended in 1978. This act specifically prohibits discrimination against persons between the ages of 40 and 70.

- The Rehabilitation Act of 1973, as amended in 1974. Again the employer is required to maintain an affirmative action program, in this case ensuring the hiring and promotion of qualified handicapped people.

- The Vietnam Era Veterans Readjustment Act of 1974. This extends the protection of affirmative action to disabled veterans and veterans of the Vietnam era employed by contractors holding federal contracts of $10,000 or more.

- Any state legislation modeled on Title VII. You should become familiar with the state equal employment opportunity acts.

Health care organizations have been the subject of court action in the area of equal pay for men and women. In the past several years, a federal district court ruled that an institution had violated the Equal Pay Act by paying its male attendants 30 cents an hour more than its female nursing aides;[7] another court decided that there was no distinction between the work performed by hospital male orderlies and female aides, and that the higher wages paid to the male orderlies were illegal under the Equal Pay Act;[8] another court declared that the job duties in a hospital for male orderlies and female nursing aides did not differ and that the higher pay scales for the orderlies was unjustified.[9] In another case, California's Fair Employment Practice Commission ruled that a hospital discriminated against a minority worker, an American Indian, when she was not rehired as a laundry worker after a leave of absence, although the hospital then employed other people for similar laundry jobs.[10]

As a supervisor doing the actual hiring, you may find yourself on the "hot seat" because of recent court decisions and settlements involving reverse discrimination. In one hospital, a suit was brought by a male private duty nurse against the hospital for not referring him for duty with female patients. The court decided that the hospital was unfairly discriminating against the male nurse and ordered the administration to reach a satisfactory agreement with the nurse regarding future assignment policy.[11]

Members of groups not included in the protected classes under various acts are beginning to test the morality of affirmative action and to question systems of quotas for protected classes. As a supervisor, you must be up-to-date on the requirements of affirmative action laws. If your institution has an affirmative action plan, review it—especially the hiring and promotion goals—to identify areas of underutilization of protected classes.

MAKING THE RIGHT CHOICE

The final decision to hire or not to hire a particular candidate should be based upon a battery of assessments. It helps to work from a planned checklist of interview findings, covering:

- *Previous experience.* Although it may not be necessary for the applicant to have exactly the experience outlined in the job description, you should consider similar job duties, similar working conditions, and the degree of supervision exercised or received on previous jobs.

- *Education and training.* You should review the candidate's formal education, major fields of study, and specialized training.

- *Manner and appearance.* You should consider general appearance, speech, nervous mannerisms, self-confidence, and aggressiveness.

- *Emotional stability and maturity.* You should consider friction with former supervisors, relationships with peers, reasons for leaving previous jobs, and job stability. You should also consider sense of responsibility and attitude toward work and toward family.

Still another checklist separates interview impressions into two areas:

1. *Personality factors.* You should determine what applicants liked best and least about their previous jobs. The answers may reveal attitudes or patterns of behavior that may be useful in evaluating applicants' suitability for the present opening. Perhaps the candidate will indicate a preference for jobs that are closely supervised or those that require independent action. Does the applicant want a job that does not demand too much or one that is routinized? Your questions should allow the applicant to reveal plans for the future. Does the candidate see this job opening as temporary or as a career commitment? Did the applicant understand each question and reply directly to the point? Was the applicant uncommunicative, or were replies responsive? Was the applicant spontaneous or more thoughtful in response to questions? Most important is consistency—was there internal agreement between the various answers and descriptions given by the candidate?

2. *Nonpersonality areas.* The candidate's educational background is important to any evaluation. Is the applicant's education adequate for the position, more than adequate, or less than adequate? Will the applicant need specific training? References should be reviewed before final evaluation. References completed by the applicant's former direct supervisors are usually the best and most accurate. It may be possible to obtain such references by telephone checks planned in advance and handled by your personnel department. Specific attention should be directed toward verifying the jobs held by the applicant, the job duties described by the applicant, and the reasons for leaving those jobs. Ask former employers whether they would rehire the applicant. In general, two specific areas

should be checked out through references: (1) the applicant's performance, and (2) the applicant's work habits, personal habits, and ability to get along with supervisors, subordinates, and fellow workers.

Pell has some cogent recommendations on evaluating an applicant and making an offer. He lists "do" and "do not" areas:

- *Do*—be specific in letters requesting references; use the telephone where possible in checking references; plan the reference interview in advance; understand the advantages and limitations of using outside investigative agencies; have realistic physical and medical standards for each position; make the job offer in person or by telephone; confirm the offer by letter.

- *Do not*—pay much attention to letters of reference carried by applicants; forget to ask a former employer why an applicant left his job; forget to ask if the company would rehire the applicant; make the job offer before reference reports are completed; accept a bad reference without question (the reference may be based on a personal dislike of the applicant by someone in the company; check it with other sources if it does not appear consistent with all other factors).[12]

Here is still another breakdown of the essential factors that make the interview effective and more scientific:

- Limit the interview to areas that cannot be measured by other methods. Tests, the application blank, and reference checks augment the interview. Remember that the interview is a public relations opportunity to market the worth of your institution.

- Train yourself in interviewing techniques. Ask your personnel department to develop an interview training seminar, or attend a seminar given by a local college or hospital or home association.

- The prime purpose of the interview is to ascertain whether the applicant would fit in with your work group and be content with the work, and whether the applicant has the qualifications to do the assigned duties.

- In the best selection programs the interview will be only one of a number of selection methods used.

- In order to be successful, the interviewer should have complete knowledge of job requirements, working conditions, and supervisory preferences before beginning the interview.[13]

KEY POINTS IN THE INTERVIEWING PROCESS

Review this list of reminders when evaluating your interviewing technique.

- Become knowledgeable about affirmative action regulations and laws.
- To match the person to the job, know in advance what the job is. Review the job description, the job specifications, and the profiles of employees who have successfully held similar jobs.
- Assemble all the information about the candidate before you start the interview. Use the application blank, the resumé (if available), references, and other preinterview information.
- Plan the interview in advance. Don't stereotype the interview. Remember to establish rapport and to communicate to the applicant complete information on the job's content and institutional policy.
- Permit time for an exchange of information, including the answering of all questions.
- Keep in mind that there are two decisions in every interview: Your decision to hire or not to hire the candidate, and the candidate's decision to accept or not to accept the position.
- Look for potential. Don't be misled by the "myth of previous experience." Look for transferable experience.
- Do not forget the candidate is under unusual stress. Do not minimize this tension, as it can affect the quality of the interview.
- Accept the fact that you are a representative of the institution, and perform a public relations function in all interviews. There is always an opportunity to make friends, even though you cannot make offers.

INTERVIEWING REVIEW PUZZLE

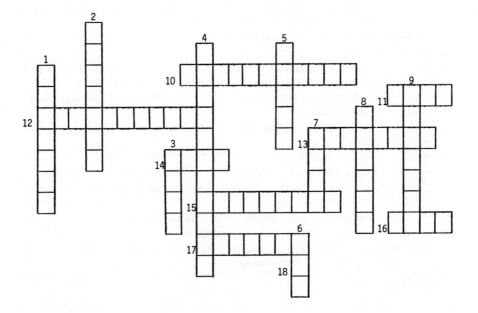

DOWN

1) Questions that are used to control the interview.
2) A type of question that is used to see if the applicant is familiar with the area being examined.
3) The interview has how many major purposes?
4) They have the final responsibility for hiring.
5) _____pay too much attention to letters of reference carried by the applicants.
6) Number of decisions to be made from the interview.
7) The interview requires a _____.
8) You should always watch your _____.
9) Plan the interview in _____.

ACROSS

10) Stage three of the interview.
11) The applicant should talk at least _____ the time.
12) Be familiar with this type of action.
13) End the interview on a _____ note.
14) The number of stages in a normal interview.
15) When there are many applicants, this type of interview is necessary.
16) Some interviewers develop quick _____.
17) You should develop this in stage one of the interview.
18) A type of useful question.

(Answers are on page 201.)

NOTES

1. Arthur R. Pell, *Recruiting and Selecting Personnel* (New York: Simon and Schuster, 1969), p. 102.

2. E.C. Webster, *Decision-Making in the Employment Interview* (Montreal: Industrial Relations Center, McGill University, 1964), pp. 13-14.

3. Pell, *Recruiting and Selecting Personnel*, p. 102.

4. Ibid., pp. 105-106.

5. N.R.S. Maier et al., *Superior-Subordinate Communications in Management, Report No. 52* (New York: American Management Association, 1961), p. 9.

6. Arthur Witkin, *Which Interviewer Are You?* (New York: Personnel Psychology Center of New York), pamphlet.

7. *Hodgson v. G. W. Hubbard Hospital of Meharry Medical College*, 351 F. Supp. 1295 (D.C., Md., Tenn., 1971).

8. *Hodgson v. Brookhaven General Hospital*, 470 F. 2d 729 (C. A. 5, 1972).

9. *Brennan v. Prince William Hospital Corporation*, 503 F. 2d 282 (C. A. 4, 1974).

10. *Northern Inyo Hospital v. Fair Employment Practice Commission*, 38 Cal. App. 3d 14 (1974).

11. *Sibley Memorial Hospital v. V. Wilson*, 488 F. 2d 1338 (C.A.D.C. 1973).

12. Pell, *Recruiting and Selecting Personnel*, pp. 150-151.

13. Milton M. Mandell, *Recruiting and Selecting Office Employees, Research Report No. 27* (New York: American Management Association, 1956), p. 73.

SUGGESTED READINGS

Basset, Glenn A. *Practical Interviewing: A Handbook for Managers*. New York: American Management Association, 1965.

Bingham, W.; Moore, B.; and Gustad, J. *How to Interview*. New York: Harper & Row, 1959.

Cannell, C.F., and Kahn, R.L. "Interviewing." In *The Handbook of Social Psychology*, edited by G. Lindzey and E. Aronson. Reading, Mass.: Addison Wesley, 1968, pp. 526-595.

Carlson, R.E.; Schwab, D.P.; and Henneman, H.G. "Agreement Among Selection Interview Styles." *Journal of Industrial Psychology* 5: 8-17.

Goyer, Robert S.; Redding, Charles W.; and Rickey, John T. *Interviewing Principles and Techniques: A Project Text*. Dubuque, Iowa: William C. Brown, 1968.

Kahn, Robert L., and Cannell, Charles F. *The Dynamics of Interviewing*. New York: John Wiley and Sons, Inc., 1964.

Mayfield, E. "The Selection Interview: A Reevaluation of Published Research." *Personnel Psychology* 17: 239-260.

Pell, Arthur R. *Recruiting and Selecting Personnel*. New York: Simon and Schuster, 1969.

Steward, C., and Cash, W. *Interviewing: Principles and Practices*. Dubuque, Iowa: William C. Brown, 1974.

Webster, E.C. *Decision-Making in the Employment Interview*. Montreal: Industrial Relations Center, McGill University, 1964.

Zima, Joseph. "Interviewing: An Imperative Interpersonal Communication Skill." In *Explorations in Speech Communication*, edited by John McKay. Columbus, Ohio: Merrill Publishing Co., 1973, pp. 91-107.

INTERVIEWING REVIEW PUZZLE

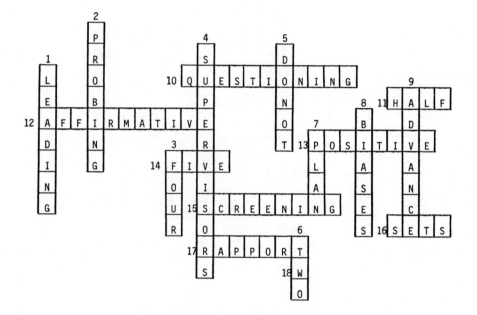

<table>
<tr><td></td><td>DOWN</td></tr>
</table>

DOWN

1) Questions that are used to control the interview.
2) A type of question that is used to see if the applicant is familiar with the area being examined.
3) The interview has how many major purposes?
4) They have the final responsibility for hiring.
5) _____ pay too much attention to letters of reference carried by the applicants.
6) Number of decisions to be made from the interview.
7) The interview requires a _____.
8) You should always watch your _____.
9) Plan the interview in _____.

ACROSS

10) Stage three of the interview.
11) The applicant should talk at least _____ the time.
12) Be familiar with this type of action.
13) End the interview on a _____ note.
14) The number of stages in a normal interview.
15) When there are many applicants, this type of interview is necessary.
16) Some interviewers develop quick _____.
17) You should develop this in stage one of the interview.
18) A type of useful question.

Chapter 11

Employee Motivation through Improved Supervision

CHAPTER OBJECTIVES

The purpose of this chapter is to enable you to CHANGE your communicative behavior in a *positive* direction. After studying the material you should be able to:

Compare your motivational needs to those of other employees.

Have an understanding of various motivational theories.

Assess your personal motivational needs and be able to rank order them in respect to their importance to *you.*

Name and employ motivational theories that are applicable to your job.

Guide yourself and your peers to meet the motivational needs of others.

Encourage *positive* thinking within your work group.

INTRODUCTION

Motivation may be thought of as an individual's ability to get people to feel, think, or act the way that individual wants them to. In other words, the person provides some type of stimuli in hopes of getting a predetermined response. Frederick Herzberg tells the following story:

> I have a year old Schnauzer. When it was a small puppy and I wanted it to move, I kicked it in the rear and it moved. Now that I have finished its obedience training, I hold up a dog biscuit when I want the Schnauzer to move. In this instance, who is motivated—I or the dog? The dog wants the biscuit, but it is I who want it to move. Again, I am the one who is motivated, and the dog is the one who moves. In this instance all I did was apply KITA (kick in the ass) frontally; I exerted a pull instead of a push. When industry wishes to use such positive KITAs, it has available an incredible number and variety of dog biscuits (jelly beans for humans) to wave in front of the employee to get him to jump.[1]

The basic premise of this chapter is that no one can motivate another. All one can hope to do is to exhibit behaviors that help others to motivate themselves. You can urge an employee to work harder, but it is the employee who must work. You cannot teach an employee a new procedure until the employee says, "Teach me, I want to learn." Most motivational theorists would agree that a supervisor's behavior, as seen by the employee, can act as a catalyst to help the employee toward self-motivation. Health care supervisors can exhibit behaviors that cause employees to behave in a particular manner and direction in order to meet a predetermined goal. H.J. Leavitt poses three basic motivational premises:

1. Behavior is caused. Things just don't happen—there are always underlying reasons.
2. Behavior is directed. In the ultimate sense, there is no aimless behavior.
3. Behavior is motivated. Underlying what we do are motives which provide us with the energy to obtain our goals or at least move in the direction of those goals.[2]

MOTIVATIONAL THEORY

Douglas McGregor has noted that theory is a most practical matter. Without underlying beliefs and assumptions we would be unable to act aside from our reflexive responses. Theory and practice are inseparable.[3]

Every time a supervisor implements a policy or action, there is a theoretic premise behind that action. Therefore, an understanding of motivational theory can enable the supervisor to respond in a reflective rather than a reflexive manner.

The early work of Abraham Maslow still serves as the main source of motivational theory today. Maslow contended that we are motivated by a hierarchy of human needs. This hierarchy takes the shape of a ladder. The first rung represents our basic need for food, clothing, and shelter. When this need is satisfied, we climb to the second rung: our need to feel safe from harm or injury. We then climb to the third rung: our need to associate with family, friends, and coworkers. The fourth rung represents our esteem needs, to be well liked, to have confidence in ourselves, and to be respected. Finally, the top rung represents self-actualization needs, the need to grow and become whatever we are capable of becoming.[4]

SELF-ACTUALIZATION
ESTEEM
BELONGINGNESS
SAFETY
BASIC NEEDS

On this ladder of basic motivational needs, we can see that we hop up and down the rungs every day of our lives. Each of these needs plays an important role in helping employees motivate themselves. However, two seem to stand out with respect to a supervisor's behavior toward a subordinate. Research indicates that most employees are motivated by supervisors who stress the belongingness and esteem needs of their employees. The organization seems to provide the basic, safety, and self-actualization needs of employees, but the responsibility to meet their belongingness and esteem needs falls upon their immediate supervisor.

Belongingness Needs

The organizational climate in Japan is centered around concepts of humanistic psychology which stipulate that human relations are just as important as production. The Japanese believe that, ultimately, the relationships between workers and management will be reflected in the quality of goods and services. They view their businesses and hospitals as social organizations, not simply as profit-oriented enterprises. The Japanese believe that the most important information flows from the bottom up, not from the top down. Their managers and supervisors expect change and initiative to come from those closest to the problem rather than from top administrators. Many American corporations are starting to shift toward this style of management.

Bob Cooper interviewed Yasuo Maetani, one of three Ajinomoto Company officials concerned with the opening of a new plant in Raleigh, North Carolina. Maetani stated:

> From a management point of view, the most important resource of the company is its human resources. Offering good pay is a primary component, but other benefits are also important. For example, the company organizes and subsidizes social activities for its workers, including tea ceremonies, flower arranging, painting and music groups, and baseball and softball teams. The management techniques of my company have paid some handsome dividends in terms of productivity in their operations. In 1978, my company embarked on a "Jump 25," a program designed to boost productivity 25 percent in three years. The goal was achieved in two. . . . Workers treat top management as members of the family, and management treats workers the same way.[5]

The service provided by your health care organization will be only as good as the people performing that service. Treat workers in an indiscriminate manner and they may treat the organization in the same way. Give them a sense of pride and a feeling that they belong, and they will perform in a more satisfied and productive way.

Esteem Needs

Esteem needs are normally defined as people's need to gain respect from their peers. However, we construct our self-esteem not only from the feedback we get from others, but also from our self-talk. The perceptions we have of different events and the words we use, in our self-talk, to interpret these events trigger pictures in our minds. These pictures (ideas) then trigger feelings that are stored subconsciously. Over time, these feelings determine how we see ourselves and, thus, how we will act under certain circumstances. Our subconscious ultimately forces us to live up or down to our self-image, which determines our level of self-esteem.

Deborah Briley believes

> . . . that individuals with low self-esteem have great difficulty in motivating themselves. Their level of self-esteem affects every aspect of their personal and professional life. People with low self-esteem lack the courage to be truthful when confronted with information that threatens their adequacy. They verbally "seduce" others with "positive strokes" in the hope that they will be "stroked" in return, which will raise their level of self-esteem. This behavior destroys their ability to do things for themselves, to make sound judgments, and their efforts ultimately end in frustration and defeat. Individuals with low self-esteem normally *use* others and cannot be loyal or devoted for any length of time. As they see themselves so do they act. And their actions tend to produce results that continually support their self-concept. If those actions are negative, their self-concept is negative resulting in low self-esteem. This chronic type of behavior perpetuates the fulfillment of their negative self-fulfilling prophesies.[6]

When supervisors are involved with employees with low self-esteem, it is imperative that they provide positive reinforcement wherever and whenever possible. People have a tendency to live up or down to labels. If employees see their supervisor holding them in high esteem, it will be much more difficult for them to fail. This does not mean they will not fail, but at least the supervisor will know that their behaviors did not contribute to that failure.

A MOTIVATIONAL SURVEY

Health care employees and supervisors at the seventh annual Hospital Topics Management Conference held in Chicago in 1979 were asked to rank certain items, first as to their importance to them personally and then as to how they thought their employees would rank them. How do you rank these items with respect to their importance to *you*? How do you think your employees would rank them? In the blank lines at the left, give each item a numerical value, one denoting the most important and five the least important in value. The results of the survey will be examined later in this chapter.

The Motivational Needs of the Health Care Professional

Your Rating	Your Employees' Rating		Supervisors' Rating	Their Employees' Rating
_____	_____	Appreciation of work done	_____	_____
_____	_____	Feeling "in" on things	_____	_____
_____	_____	Professional growth	_____	_____
_____	_____	Challenging work	_____	_____
_____	_____	Good wages	_____	_____

Appreciation of Work Done

The perceptions of health care employees are extremely important. Whatever they believe to be true is true for them. If they feel they are part of a team, they are indeed part of a team. Individuals can respond to appreciation of work done only in terms of their perceptions. Therefore, the result of communication between supervisor and subordinate will be what the subordinate perceives it to be.

Elton Mayo conducted a series of experiments at the Hawthorne plant of the Western Electric Company near Chicago. The experiments were primarily concerned with the effect of working conditions on worker productivity. One of the hypotheses concerned the relationship between production and lighting intensity in the plant. Mayo did not find the relationship he expected, but he was amazed at what he did discover. He noticed that even when the lights were practically turned off, worker production increased. This classic result became known as the Hawthorne effect. The increase in production was attributed to the fact that the workers were receiving attention, even when working conditions deteriorated as a result of this attention.[7]

The Hawthorne effect strongly suggests that the workers perceived the study's attention as a form of caring, as an indication of management wanting to improve conditions for the workers because they were important to the organization.

A hospital dietician stated it this way: "I'm a part of the health care team. I want to be appreciated. If a dietician and an endocrinologist are working together with a diabetic patient, and the diabetic is well managed and adheres to a diet, then the patient may not need insulin."

We all want to feel that what we do counts, that we can make a difference. Do you notice a positive change in the morale of your employees after they attend a convention or training seminar? Only when workers improve their attitudes and skills will the organization improve.

Feeling "in" on Things

Employees at times become irked at the indifferent attitudes shown by supervisors toward work-related problems. This type of demeaning supervision can be humiliating for the employee, can stop the flow of feedback from the supervisor, and inhibit the employee's ability to participate in the decision-making process.

W.C. Redding found that good communication characterizes effective managerial leadership:

- The better supervisors tend to be communication-minded, are able to explain instructions and policies, and enjoy conversing with subordinates.

- The better supervisors tend to be empathic listeners; they respond understandingly to "silly" questions; they are approachable; they will listen to suggestions and complaints with an attitude of fair consideration and a willingness to take appropriate action.

- The better supervisors tend to ask or persuade rather than tell or demand.

- The better supervisors tend to be sensitive to the feelings and ego-defense needs of their subordinates; they are careful to reprimand in private rather than in public.

- The better supervisors openly pass along information; they give advance notice of impending changes and supply "reasons" for policies and regulations.[8]

When employees are not involved in the decision-making process and are rarely consulted, there is a tendency to let down and not be totally involved in the job. The result of such indifference is job dissatisfaction. It follows that, if employees feel they are not wisely utilized, it is next to impossible to instill any degree of pride into their work. High job satisfaction and quality work depend upon the maximum use of the individual worker's training and skill.

Employees can be motivated only through the sharing of power, not through the exertion of power by a supervisor. Sometimes supervisors exert tremendous pressure on obstinate employees. Robert N. Ford tells us that "the obstinate employee is trying to tell us something. . . it's not recognize me as implied by the Hawthorne studies, nor treat me well . . . the employee is saying use me well. Let my life mean something."[9]

F.B. Chaney discovered that there was a positive correlation between performance and job attitude and the degree of participation in the decision-making process. He reported zero improvement for people in no-participation to low-participation groups, while the high-participation groups showed an attitude and production improvement of 80 percent and 95 percent, respectively.[10]

If there is a work-related problem in your group, rather than have one individual try to solve it, why not call the group together to share ideas? No one knows the job better than the individual employees who are doing it day in and day out.

Professional Growth

Work must be a source of personal enrichment; employees must feel that they have an opportunity to grow and become the professionals they are capable of becoming. Participating in in-house training programs, attending conventions, and belonging to professional organizations help the employee fulfill the needs of self-actualization.

Frederick Herzberg examined factors affecting job attitudes. He tallied 1,844 events on the job that, when absent, led to extreme dissatisfaction. He labeled these events *maintenance factors*. These maintenance factors created job dissatisfaction only when they were absent from the job. He also tallied 1,753 events on the job that led to extreme satisfaction. These he called *motivators*.

Herzberg, like Maslow, found that motivational needs are not mutually exclusive, that indeed one may build upon the other. Also, people may be motivated by several needs at the same time.

Herzberg rank ordered the following motivators and maintenance factors by their percentage of frequency:[11]

Motivators	*Maintenance Factors*
Extreme Satisfaction	*Extreme Dissatisfaction*
1. Achievement	1. Company policy and administration
2. Recognition	2. Supervision
3. Work itself	3. Relationship with supervisor
4. Responsibility	4. Work conditions
5. Advancement	5. Salary
6. Growth	6. Relationship with peers

It appears from this that workers, more than ever before, are seeking self-fulfillment, self-development, and the enhancement of life through the quality of their work.

Challenging Work

Employees are increasingly concerned about two themes: (1) concern that the job be a source of personal fulfillment, and (2) the right to assert individual rights on the job, sometimes called the "psychology of entitlement." When employees feel that they are a part of a team working toward a common goal, their level of personal fulfillment will be raised. When their questions and suggestions are listened to, their individual rights as professionals are maintained. Today, worker values are shifting. The baby-boom children who came into the job force in the late sixties and early seventies account for this new youthfulness. Employees under 30 years of age are demanding that a job be both interesting and challenging. Older employees are now starting to express this same sentiment. They want to feel that what they do matters. There is greater demand to be heard and to be involved in the decision-making process.

When employees feel dissatisfied, it is usually because they feel they are not being wisely utilized based on their experience and training. Supervisors should ask themselves if a particular job makes the maximum use of an employee's abilities. Today, it takes more than money to motivate employees. The motivational needs of employees are changing as rapidly as technology. These needs must be met if employees are to be expected to motivate themselves.

Good Wages

Money will initially attract people to a particular career or job, but most motivational theorists will tell you that money is not a long-lasting motivator. Workers quickly forget about that raise they received six months ago. Employees like to complain about low wages, about their pay not keeping up with inflation. But sometimes the reasons for complaining run deeper than merely low wages. It could be that they are unhappy about other aspects of their jobs, or they may feel that, if they don't complain, their raises won't be very good. One of the basic reasons for such dissatisfaction, however, may be that they think, or they find out, that they are not earning as much money as others with equal skills and training. If employees are making salaries similar to those of other employees in the same geographical area and with equal years of experience, money will not be the primary issue.

Merrill Lynch Relocation Management Incorporated, which specializes in moving executives, estimates that 200,000 to 300,000 executives will be asked by their employers to move to new locations but that one-third to one-half of them will refuse, even though the move means higher rank and pay. Only a decade ago, the refusal rate was less than ten percent.[12]

The University of Michigan Survey Research Center asked 1,553 working people to rank order various aspects of their jobs in order of importance. The center discovered that "good pay" came in fifth behind "interesting work," "enough help and equipment to get the job done," "enough information to do the job," and "enough authority to do the job."[13]

Results of the Motivational Survey

Earlier in this chapter, you were asked to rank order five factors pertaining to the motivational needs of the health care professional (note the similarity between that survey and the University of Michigan survey just cited). In the initial survey, supervisors were asked to rank order the items with respect to their importance to them personally. They were then asked to rank the items with respect to how they thought their employees would rank them. The purpose was to determine if management had an accurate perception of what was *really* important to employees from a motivational point of view. The results (compared with your rankings to the left) are shown in the two right-hand columns below.

Your Rating	Your Employees' Rating		Supervisors' Rating	Their Employees' Rating
_____	_____	Appreciation of work done	1	4
_____	_____	Feeling "in" on things	2	5
_____	_____	Professional growth	3	2
_____	_____	Challenging work	4	3
_____	_____	Good wages	5	1

Several generalizations can be made from this study. The study seems to suggest that employees do want to be involved in their jobs. When they become less involved, their job satisfaction decreases. Consequently, they become dissatisfied with the organization. Low employee morale translates into employee turnover and/or absenteeism, which results in lost revenue. When an employee is absent, someone else must do that employee's job. To eliminate this problem it is important that the motivational needs of employees be met.

It is much easier to communicate in a meaningful manner if we have a data base from which to draw conclusions about one another's motivational needs. Only through congruent perceptions can we solve problems and work together toward a common goal. Too many times our perceptions of another's needs are false perceptions. For example, if money is important to us, we assume it's important to others as well. Therefore, we don't take the time or effort to seek genuine feedback. Many times, hospital policy is based on inaccurate information; and, to compound the problem, when employees are asked for feedback, they sometimes fail to be open and honest and they supply faulty information, disguising the real issues.

Many different types of instruments are used in an attempt to determine organizational and employee needs. The feedback information from such instruments can be used to implement new policies or, if need be, to change existing ones.

The following Motivation Feedback Questionnaire will tell you what motivates you. However, remember that, just because some of these items motivate you, that does not mean they will motivate everyone else. A popular television show had the theme, "Different Strokes for Different Folks." With respect to motivational theory, that theme holds true.

Motivation Feedback Questionnaire
Part I

Directions:
The following statements have seven possible responses.

Strongly agree	Agree	Slightly agree	Don't know	Slightly disagree	Disagree	Strongly disagree
+3	+2	+1	0	−1	−2	−3

Please score each statement by circling the number that corresponds to your response. For example, if you "strongly agree," circle the number +3.

1. Special salary increases should be given to employees who do their jobs well. +3 +2 +1 0 −1 −2 −3

2. Better job descriptions would be helpful so that employees know exactly what is expected of them. +3 +2 +1 0 −1 −2 −3

3. Employees need to be reminded that their jobs are dependent upon the group's ability to meet its objective. +3 +2 +1 0 −1 −2 −3

4. Supervisors should give a great deal of attention to the physical working conditions of their employees. +3 +2 +1 0 −1 −2 −3

5. Supervisors ought to work hard to develop a friendly working atmosphere among their employees. +3 +2 +1 0 −1 −2 −3

6. Individual recognition for above-standard performance means a lot to employees. +3 +2 +1 0 −1 −2 −3

7. Indifferent supervision can often bruise feelings. +3 +2 +1 0 −1 −2 −3

8. Employees want to feel that their real skills and capacities are put to use on their jobs. +3 +2 +1 0 −1 −2 −3

9. The group's retirement benefits and medical insurance programs are important factors in keeping employees on their jobs. +3 +2 +1 0 −1 −2 −3

10. Almost every job can be made more stimulating and challenging. +3 +2 +1 0 −1 −2 −3

11. Many employees want to give their best in everything they do. +3 +2 +1 0 −1 −2 −3

12. Management could show more interest in the employees by sponsoring social events after hours. +3 +2 +1 0 −1 −2 −3

13. Pride in one's work is actually an important reward. +3 +2 +1 0 −1 −2 −3

14. Employees want to think of themselves as the "best" at their jobs. +3 +2 +1 0 −1 −2 −3

15.	The quality of the relationship in the informal work group is quite important.	+3 +2 +1	0 −1 −2 −3
16.	Individual merit raises would improve the performance of employees.	+3 +2 +1	0 −1 −2 −3
17.	Visibility with upper management is important to employees.	+3 +2 +1	**0** −1 −2 −3
18.	Employees generally like to schedule their own work and make job-related decisions with a minimum of supervision.	+3 +2 +1	0 −1 −2 −3
19.	Job security is important to employees.	+3 +2 +1	0 −1 −2 −3
20.	Having good equipment to work with is important to employees.	+3 +2 +1	0 −1 −2 −3

Part II

Scoring:
1. Enter the numbers you circled in Part I in the blanks below after the appropriate statement number.

Statement No.	Score		Statement No.	Score
10	___		2	___
11	___		3	___
13	___		9	___
18	___		19	___
Self-Actualization	___ Total		Safety	___ Total

Statement No.	Score		Statement No.	Score
6	___		1	___
8	___		4	___
14	___		16	___
17	___		20	___
Esteem	___ Total		Basic	___ Total

Statement No.	Score
5	___
7	___
12	___
15	___
Belongingness	___ Total

2. Record your scores in the chart by putting an "X" in each row under the number of your total score for that area of need-motivation. After you have completed this chart, you can see the relative strength of your response in each area of "need-motivation." There is of course no "right" answer. What motivates you might not motivate someone else. In general, however, most motivational theorists believe that most employees are motivated by managers who stress the belongingness and esteem needs of their employees.

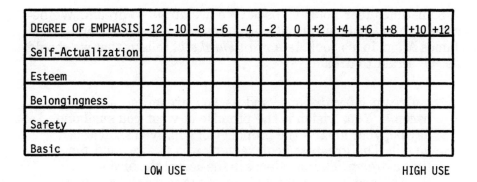

DEGREE OF EMPHASIS	-12	-10	-8	-6	-4	-2	0	+2	+4	+6	+8	+10	+12
Self-Actualization													
Esteem													
Belongingness													
Safety													
Basic													

LOW USE   HIGH USE

POSITIVE THINKING

If there is one trait that separates average human beings from exceptional ones, it is that exceptional human beings talk positively to themselves. They are optimistic rather than pessimistic.

Jim Valvano, head basketball coach at North Carolina State University, explains the difference between the two:

> Two brothers are opening their Christmas presents. The first boy unwrapped a beautiful, shiny electric car. But he didn't seem happy and his father asked him what was the matter. "Well," he said, "I'm afraid the battery might run down and the car won't run and you would be mad at me."
> The second boy opened his package and found manure. He acted real excited and started throwing it in all directions. The father told him there had been a mistake, but wondered why he had been so pleased. The boy said, "There must be a pony in here someplace."[14]

The exceptional person holds himself in high esteem and is *not* afraid to dream. It has been said that dreamers are the saviors of the world. Successful organizations have a way of coping with problems by implementing new equipment or ideas that were at one time just dreams. Yet someone had the self-confidence, enthusiasm, and the desire to work in order to make the dreams come true. Nothing is ever accomplished without enthusiasm, but effort is also necessary. Together, they are an unbeatable combination.

Sometimes fear holds us back. We are afraid to dream. We become cynics, distrustful not only of others but also of ourselves. James Allen, in his book *As A Man Thinketh,* tells us that we should not be afraid to dream:

> Dream lofty dreams, and as you dream, so shall you become. Your vision is the promise of what you shall one day be; your ideal is the prophecy of what you shall at last unveil. The greatest achievement was at first and for a time a dream. The oak sleeps in the acorn; the bird waits in the egg; and in the highest vision of the soul a waking angel stirs. Dreams are the seedlings of realities. . . . Into your hands will be placed the exact results of your own thoughts; you will receive that which you earn; no more, no less. Whatever your present environment may be, you will fall, remain, or rise with your thoughts, your Vision, your Ideal.[15]

The late Bo Rein was head football coach at North Carolina State University from 1975 to 1980. During that time, he took his team to two bowl games and one Atlantic Coast Conference championship. Before every team meal and before every game, he had his players recite the following prayer. The prayer not only has spiritual implications but also stresses the need for positive thinking, enthusiasm, work, and dedication:

What Will Today Bring?

> This is the beginning of a new day.
> God has given me this day to use as I will.
> I can waste it or use it for good.
> What I do today is important, because I'm exchanging
>   a day of my life for it.
> When tomorrow comes this day will be gone forever,
>   ieaving in its place something I have traded for it.
> I want it to be gain, not loss; good, not evil;
>   success, not failure; in order that I shall not
>   regret the price I paid for it because the future
>   is just a whole string of nows.[16]

Health care supervisors should remember that it is easy to think positively when things are going well but much more difficult when everything seems to be going wrong. When things go wrong, one should remember that "the sun never shines on the same dog." At such times, positive thinkers will call upon a deep inner strength to overcome what to some would be the insurmountable. Positive thinkers know that there are no limits, no constraints, within the laws of common decency that will limit or defeat them in accomplishing their goals.

A FINAL SAFEGUARD

However, the positive thinker must constantly be on guard to avoid developing a Machiavellian attitude, a tendency to manipulate others. This personality variable plays an important role in our lives. All of us have at times exhibited Machiavellian tendencies. Supervisors thus should be aware of high Machiavellian ("high-Mach") attitudes in their own behaviors and in the behaviors of others. A person with high-Mach believes that the end *always* justifies the means. Such a person says, "If you want it, go for it," but fails to recognize that normally "we get what we deserve."

High-Mach individuals take stock of a situation, rationally calculate their own advantage, manipulate people to their own ends, treat them as pawns or as things, and do not feel bound by the moral beliefs of others. They do not hesitate to use force or fraud to accomplish their selfish goals.[17] They never tell anyone the real reason they did something unless the telling is useful to them. They believe it is wise to flatter important people.[18] Finally, though they are entirely amoral in their outlook, when they are the victim of some transgression they become highly indignant; in such cases, they, the victimizers, blame the victim.[19]

The goals you set for yourself and your work group must depend upon truth through open and honest communication. There must be no room for Machiavellianism. Once a group decision is made, individuals cannot keep changing it, as new circumstances arise, just to meet their own selfish personal needs. Positive thinking requires a sharing of positive thoughts through and with others. What affects you will affect others. The sharing of dreams, hopes, wishes, and frustrations moves you and others closer toward the accomplishment of a common goal. Sharing through positive thinking is a two-way process.

Sometimes when we think we have lost, we really have won. There will be times when our hopes and our dreams do not materialize in the manner we had envisioned. At such times, we may look upon the situation as hopeless and fail to see the advantages that can accrue from a lost cause. It is at times like this that information must be honestly shared. This sharing must be a gain, not a loss, a good, not an evil, so that you and your work group will not regret the price you have paid for ultimate success. Positive thinkers must constantly remind themselves that the glass is never half empty—it is always half full.

MOTIVATION REVIEW PUZZLE

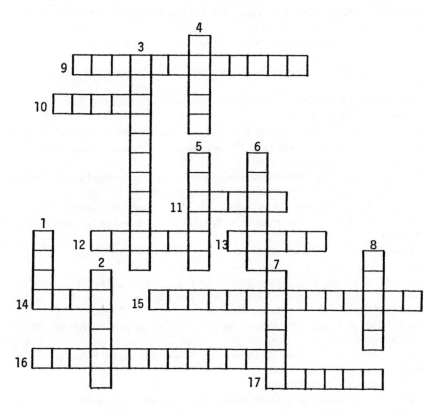

DOWN

1) Who motivates you?
2) Ranked third by employees.
3) Creates extreme satisfaction.
4) How employees rated good wages.
5) The primary concern of a hospital.
6) Developed hierarchy of human needs.
7) To respect.
8) A long-lasting motivator.

ACROSS

9) Employees rank it number one.
10) Need for food, clothing, and shelter.
11) Improves morale.
12) Their responses determine quality of service.
13) Is not a long-lasting motivator.
14) Few people are motivated by this.
15) Improves morale.
16) What decision making should be.
17) You want a high degree of this.

(Answers are on page 224.)

NOTES

1. Frederick Herzberg, "One More Time: How Do You Motivate Employees?" *Harvard Business Review* 46, no. 1: 53-62.

2. H.J. Leavitt, *Managerial Psychology* (Chicago: University of Chicago Press, 1972), pp. 5-10.

3. Douglas McGregor, *The Human Side of Enterprise* (New York: McGraw-Hill Book Co., 1960), p. 6.

4. Abraham Maslow, *Motivation and Personality* (New York: Harper & Row, 1954).

5. *Raleigh Times*, May 29, 1980.

6. Deborah Briley, in a round-table discussion, Cary, North Carolina, March 27, 1980.

7. Gerald M. Goldhaber, *Organizational Communication* (Dubuque, Iowa: William C. Brown Co., Publishers, 1979), p. 40.

8. W.C. Redding, *Communication Within the Organization* (West Lafayette, Ind.: Purdue University, Industrial Communications Council, 1972), p. 443.

9. Robert N. Ford, "The Obstinate Employee," *Public Opinion Quarterly* 24: 301-310.

10. F.B. Chaney, "Employee Participation in Manufacturing Job Design," *Human Factors* 11: 101-106.

11. Herzberg, "One More Time," pp. 53-62.

12. *Time*, June 12, 1978.

13. Donald M. Morrison, "Is the Work Ethic Going Out of Style?" in *The Challenge of the Future: Visions and Versions*, ed. Bill Conboy (Lawrence, Kans.: University of Kansas, Division of Continuing Education, 1979), p. 161.

14. Jim Valvano, at a sales rally held by Carolina Partners of Raleigh, Raleigh, North Carolina, April, 1980.

15. James Allen, *As A Man Thinketh* (New York: Grosset and Dunlap Publishers, 1978), pp. 59-63.

16. Bo Rein; personal communication.

17. Stanley S. Guterman, *The Machiavellians* (Lincoln, Nebr.: University of Nebraska Press, 1970), pp. vii-viii.

18. Ibid., pp. 3-4.

19. Ibid., p. 39.

SUGGESTED READINGS

Atkinson, J.W., and Raynor, J.O. *Motivation and Achievement*. New York: Halstead Press, 1974.

Beer, M. *Leadership, Employee Needs, and Motivation*. Columbus, Ohio : Bureau of Business Research, Ohio State University, 1966.

Bennett, Addison C. "Effective Management Centers on Human Values." *Hospitals, JAHA*, July 16, 1976, pp. 73-75.

Centers, R., and Bugental, D. "Intrinsic and Extrinsic Motivations Among Different Segments of the Working Population." *Journal of Applied Psychology* 50: 193-197.

Dalton, Gene W., and Lawrence, Paul R. *Motivation and Control in Organizations*. Homewood, Ill.: Richard D. Irwin, Inc., 1971.

Evans, M. "Herzberg's Two Factor Motivation: Some Problems and a Suggested Test." *Personnel Journal* 49: 32-35.

Gellerman, Saul W. *Motivation and Productivity*. New York: American Management Association, 1963.

Goble, Frank. *The Third Force: The Psychology of Abraham Maslow*. New York: Grossman Publishers, 1970.

Hall, D.T., and Nougaim, K.E., "An Examination of Maslow's Need Hierarchy in An Organizational Setting." *Organizational Behavior and Human Performance* 5, no. 1: 12-35.

Herzberg, Frederick. "One More Time: How Do You Motivate Employees?" *Harvard Business Review* 46, no. 1: 53-62.

———. *Work and the Nature of Man*. New York: The World Publishing Company, 1966.

House, R.J., and Wingdor, L.A. "Herzberg's Dual-Factor Theory of Job Satisfaction and Motivation." *Personal Psychology* 20, no. 4: 369-389.

Likert, Rensis. *Motivation: The Core of Management, Personnel Series No. 155*. New York: American Management Association, 1953, pp. 3-20.

Maslow, Abraham H. *Motivation and Personality*. New York: Harper & Row, 1970.

———. *Toward A Psychology of Being*. Princeton, N.J.: Van Nostrand Insight Books, 1968.

McClelland, David C., ed. *Studies in Motivation*. New York: Appleton-Century-Crofts, 1955.

McGregor, Douglas. *Leadership and Motivation*. Edited by Warren G. Bennis and Edgar H. Schien. Cambridge, Mass.: Massachusetts Institute of Technology Press, 1966.

Moser, George V. "How Not to Influence People." *Management Record*, March 1958.

Schneider, Frank W., and Delaney, James D. "Effect of Individual Achievement Motivation on Group Problem Solving Efficiency." *Journal of Social Psychology* 86: 291-298.

Steers, Richard M., and Porter, Lyman, W. *Motivation and Work Behavior*. New York: McGraw-Hill Book Co., 1975.

Vroom, Victor H. *Work and Motivation*. New York: John Wiley and Sons, Inc., 1964.

MOTIVATION REVIEW PUZZLE

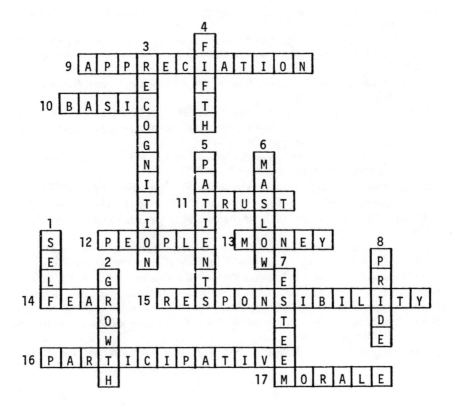

DOWN

1) Who motivates you?
2) Ranked third by employees.
3) Creates extreme satisfaction.
4) How employees rated good wages.
5) The primary concern of a hospital.
6) Developed hierarchy of human needs.
7) To respect.
8) A long-lasting motivator.

ACROSS

9) Employees rank it number one.
10) Need for food, clothing, and shelter.
11) Improves morale.
12) Their responses determine quality of service.
13) Is not a long-lasting motivator.
14) Few people are motivated by this.
15) Improves morale.
16) What decision making should be.
17) You want a high degree of this.

Supervisors' Checklist: It's Time to Take Inventory*

*The authors wish to acknowledge the work of Dr. Leslie M. Slote, industrial psychologist, Hartsdale, N.Y., who developed many of these suggestions for supervisory practices at the various levels.

CHECKLIST A: FOR DEPARTMENT-HEAD LEVEL

This soul-searching exercise is directed toward key management personnel in health care facilities who are responsible for entire departments and, therefore, have other levels of supervision reporting to them. It is a review of some of the material covered earlier and some of the questions posed. It is a good idea to ask yourself these questions periodically throughout the year.

1. Do you as a department head set the pace and attitudes for your people?
2. Do your people share the job of developing goals?
3. Do you share with your people the goals of the institution?
4. Do you give your people a sense of direction, something to strive for and achieve?
5. Does each member of your department understand the relationship and importance of his or her individual job to the department's operations and to the institution's operations?
6. Do the people in your department understand their responsibilities?
7. Do you endorse the management theory that if subordinates are to plan their course intelligently and work efficiently they need to know the where, what, and why of their jobs: where they are going, what they are doing, and why they are doing it?
8. Do your subordinates have a feeling of being "in" on things?
9. Do you share information or do you keep secrets?
10. Are the supervisors who report to you familiar with top management's thinking, the latest institutional-wide developments, and the relative importance of various departmental activities to the institution's short- and long-range plans?
11. Do you recognize and accept that it is your responsibility and a priority obligation to keep everyone in your department informed of institutional policy, day-to-day decisions, and most important, reasons for change that affect them as individuals and as work groups?
12. Do your supervisors understand and accept the institution's goals and know how to motivate their subordinates to achieve those goals?
13. Do you notify your people ahead of time of impending changes?

14. Do your requests to your subordinates include the reasons for the requests?
15. Do you have an accurate feedback mechanism?
16. Do you know how your people react to your decisions?
17. Do you know how your people perceive you and the administration?
18. Are you able to cope with rapidly changing situations?
19. Are you able to replan, reorganize, and take emergency action when indicated?
20. Do you have confidence in the people who work for you?
21. Do you indicate such confidence by delegating responsibility with appropriate authority?
22. Are your actions consistent?
23. Are your actions predictable?
24. Do you recognize effort and good work?
25. Do you recognize poor effort and attempt to correct it promptly?
26. Are you convinced that it is just as easy to be positive as to be negative?
27. Do you realize that praise and encouragement often are more productive than criticism?
28. Do your employees feel free to bring problems to you?
29. Have you established a receptive atmosphere for hearing and acting on employee complaints and suggestions?
30. Are you developing understudies from your immediate management level?
31. Is there someone in the department who can replace you if you leave?
32. Do you have a carefully considered supervisory selection and training program for obtaining and developing the type of supervision you want?
33. Do you hold a good person down in one position because he or she is so indispensable there?
34. Do you take a chance on your people by letting them learn through mistakes, by showing a calm reaction and constructive approach to occasional failure, by encouraging them to stick their necks out without fear of the ax, and by instilling self-confidence?
35. Do you use every opportunity to build up in subordinates a sense of the importance of their work?
36. Are you giving real responsibility to your immediate supervisors and then holding them accountable?

37. Do you interfere with jobs of subordinates or do you allow them to exercise discretion and judgment in making decisions?
38. Are you doing things to discourage your subordinates?
39. Are you interested in and aware of the sources of discontentment, or discouragement, or frustration affecting your supervisors?
40. Do you encourage and listen to the ideas and reactions of your subordinates?
41. Do you give your subordinates credit for their contributions?
42. Do you explain to them why their ideas or suggestions are not acceptable?
43. Do you remember to praise in public but criticize in private?
44. Are you aware that a feeling of belonging builds self-confidence and makes people want to work harder than ever?
45. Do you show your people a future?
46. Are you aware of the fact that maximum self-development always takes place when a person feels, understands, accepts, and exercises the full weight of responsibility for his or her job?

CHECKLIST B: FOR INTERMEDIATE-LEVEL SUPERVISORS

You are in a position where you report to a department head and have first-line supervisors reporting to you. Refer to this checklist throughout the year to gauge your effectiveness.

1. Do you have a thorough understanding of institutional goals, your part in meeting budgets, and do you have full confidence in their attainment?
2. Do you offer suggestions or constructive criticism to your supervisor (the department head) and ask for additional information when necessary?
3. Do you build team spirit and group pride by getting everyone into the act of setting goals and pulling together?
4. Do you deal with emergencies as they come up or do you have scheduled times for meetings with your department head and with your first-line supervisors?
5. Do you encourage each of your supervisors to come up with suggestions on ways to improve things?

6. When you do not accept your supervisors' suggestions, do you explain why?
7. Have you set up an atmosphere that enables your subordinates to approach you with job or personal problems?
8. Do people believe that you listen empathetically and really care about their problems?
9. Do you keep your supervisors informed on how they are doing?
10. Do you give credit where credit is due and offer constructive criticism when necessary?
11. Do your supervisors appear to be too busy with work problems to be concerned about their employees' personal difficulties?
12. Does your example encourage your supervisors to build individual worker confidence and praise good performance?
13. Do your supervisors know that you expect them to communicate to their people how jobs are evaluated and what the job rates and progressions are?
14. Do your supervisors keep their people informed of promotional opportunities?
15. Do your supervisors train their people for better jobs?

CHECKLIST C: FOR IMMEDIATE/FIRST-LINE SUPERVISORS

As a first-line supervisor, you should review the following checklist on a regular basis.

1. Do you know that good communication means being available to answer employee questions?
2. Do you accept employees' need to know what is expected of them, how well they are doing their jobs, and how they will be rewarded for good work?
3. Have you permitted your employees freedom and latitude in performing their work, or are you constantly supervising employees?
4. Are you personally interested in the well-being of the people who work for you?
5. Do you recommend good workers for promotions, merit increases, and other forms of recognition?
6. Do you consult with your employees and permit them to share in the decision-making process?

7. Do you realize that pent-up emotions are dangerous and, therefore, do you provide an accessible sounding board for employee complaints and grievances?
8. Do you ever say or do anything that detracts from the sense of personal dignity that each of your people has?
9. When a job is well done do you praise the worker; and when a job is done poorly do you criticize constructively?
10. Do you realize that people want to feel important?
11. Do you realize that people want recognition?
12. Do you realize that people want credit and attention?
13. Do you realize that people have their own self-interest at heart?
14. Do you realize that people want to be better off tomorrow than today?
15. Do you realize that people want prompt action on their questions?
16. Do you realize that people would rather talk than listen?
17. Do you realize that people would rather give advice than take advice?
18. Do you realize that people generally resent too-close supervision?
19. Do you realize that people resent change?
20. Do you realize that people are naturally curious?
21. Do you ask questions instead of giving orders?
22. Do you make suggestions instead of giving orders?
23. Do you keep in mind the employees' self-interest?
24. Do you make your employees feel that their work is useful?
25. Do you make your employees feel that they are trusted members of the work group?
26. Do you represent your employees' interests to the next level of supervision?
27. Do you represent the management to your employees?
28. Are you too busy with work problems to be concerned with employees' personal difficulties?
29. Do you look for and find opportunities to praise and reward a good performance, or are you afraid of being accused of sentimentality and coddling?
30. Are you consistent, or do you play favorites?
31. Are you predictable, or do your employees feel they never know what your next move will be?
32. Do you try to rotate your people and build up skills for individual flexibility within the group?

33. Do you spend enough time training your people?
34. Do you understand the problem with legislating change rather than selling change?
35. Do your employees perceive you as a "people-centered" supervisor?
36. Do your employees trust you?

Appendix B
Supervisor Evaluation

SUPERVISION EVALUATION

Would you dare ask your employees to complete this survey rating you as a supervisor? How would you rate yourself?

1. Supervisor's relationship with his/her staff: Well liked and respected ( ), Usually gets along well with others and makes fair impression ( ), Seldom attracts respect from others ( ), Creates antagonism ( ).
2. Work knowledge of supervisor: Excellent ( ), Good ( ), Fair ( ), I know more than him/her ( ).
3. Does he/she set a good example? Always ( ), Sometimes ( ), If I used him/her as an example I'd be fired ( ).
4. Does he/she provide motivation?   Yes ( ) No ( )
5. Do you receive respect?   Yes ( ) No ( )
6. Are you dealt with honestly?   Yes ( ) No ( )
7. Do you receive praise on a job well done?   Yes ( ) No ( )
8. Are you criticized when you perform poorly? Yes ( ) No ( )
   Is this criticism beneficial?   Yes ( ) No ( )
9. Are you encouraged to take initiative?   Yes ( ) No ( )
10. Are you encouraged to make suggestions?   Yes ( ) No ( )
11. Is your supervisor too demanding?   Yes ( ) No ( )
12. Are schedules and job assignments made
    fairly?   Yes ( ) No ( )
13. Do you feel your supervisor plays
    favorites?   Yes ( ) No ( )
14. Do you feel you were adequately oriented
    to your job?   Yes ( ) No ( )
15. Do you feel your supervisor is willing to
    help with work if your team is shorthanded? Yes ( ) No ( )
16. Do you feel your supervisor has a heavy
    work load?   Yes ( ) No ( )
17. If you want to speak with your supervisor
    will he/she find the time?   Yes ( ) No ( )
18. Do you feel your supervisor will listen
    with an open mind?   Yes ( ) No ( )
19. Does your supervisor accept criticism?   Yes ( ) No ( )
20. Do you feel lines of communication are
    open above your supervisor?   Yes ( ) No ( )
21. Do unresolved problems with your super-
    visor reflect on his/her attitude toward
    you?   Yes ( ) No ( )

22. Are problems usually worked out?   Yes ( ) No ( )
23. Do you feel your supervisor will stand
    behind you when you are right?   Yes ( ) No ( )
24. Do you feel your supervisor cares about
    your personal feelings and problems?   Yes ( ) No ( )

Appendix C

Programmed
Chapter Review

This appendix contains a programmed chapter review of the material covered in the book. The answers are in the column to the left of the questions. Cover the answers with a note card and lower the card after you answer each question. If you give an incorrect response, go back and review the appropriate chapter before continuing with the review:

CHAPTER 1—HOW TO COMMUNICATE FOR CHANGE

change	1.	If there is a single consistency in today's complex health care industry, it is the move toward _____ .
resistant	2.	No matter what the change may be, the average employee will be suspicious and often _____ .
insignificant	3.	To the employee in your department, there is no such thing as an _____ change.
predicted	4.	Many a supervisor has made a new process turn out to be just as impractical as the supervisor _____ it would be.
norms, customs	5.	Use group _____ and _____ in planning and implementing change.
detail	6.	It is essential that the reasons for the change be communicated in _____ .
communication	7.	Good _____ is essential to good employee relations.
downward	8.	A _____ flow of formal communications is typical of most institutions.
listening	9.	In all communication, _____ is just as important as talking.
meaning	10.	Words do not have _____ within themselves.
Feedback	11.	_____ should be considered a way of giving help.
evaluative	12.	Feedback should not be _____ .
cooperation	13.	More often than not, change requires _____ .
appreciation	14.	The need for _____ stands at the top of the pyramid of employee "wants."
cooperate	15.	It is just not possible to force people to _____ .
consensus	16.	Decisions reached by _____ have enormous positive effects on productivity.

communication

17. No matter how varied your activities may be and how specialized your skills are, in the final analysis your success as a supervisor is related to _____ .

want

18. Your subordinates often tell you what they think you _____ to hear.

trust, confidence

19. If you want to obtain accurate information, you must develop an organizational style based on _____ and _____ .

vacuum

20. You never communicate in a _____ .

sender, receiver

21. No matter what form communication takes, there is a _____ and a _____ .

downward, horizontal

22. Communication should be thought of as directional—upward, _____ , or _____ from the sender.

not

23. One cannot _____ communicate.

repetition

24. Although many supervisors feel that a message should be transmitted only once, specialists insist that _____ is important.

received, fidelity

25. Communication does not occur merely because a message is sent; it must also be _____ with reasonable _____ .

CHAPTER 2—THE SUPERVISOR AS AN ORGANIZATIONAL CLIMATE MAKER

perception

26. William Evans defined organizational climate as a multidimensional _____ by members as well as nonmembers of the essential attributes or character of an organizational system.

behavioral

27. Perceptions of organizational climate, whether real or unreal, have _____ consequences for the organization.

similar
different

28. Organizational climate is both _____ to and _____ from the weather.

see, touch
sense

29. Organizational climate is not something that we can directly _____ or _____, but we can nevertheless _____ it.

environment
change

30. People create their own work _____; if it isn't right, people can _____ it.

high

31. Numerous studies have shown that certain types of climates typify _____ performance groups.

behavior	32. The _____ a supervisor exhibits on the job helps to determine the organizational climate.
highly	33. K.W. Back discovered that _____ cohesive
communication	groups tend to place more value on _____
low	than groups of _____ cohesion.
six	34. There are _____ climate dimensions that can
two	be classified into _____ groups.
aspiration	35. Alvin Zander found that a group's _____ level helps to determine its degree of success or failure.
	36. Cartwright discovered that members of cohe-
influence	sive groups tend to exert more _____ over one another and are more readily influenced by
noncohesive	one another, compared to members of _____ groups.
	37. When joining a group, a person employs a
comparison	standard called the _____ level.
trust, performance	38. High _____ tends to stimulate high _____ and increase employee confidence, loyalty, and teamwork.
	39. Highly motivated individuals tend to work in
supportive	_____ organizational climates.
climates	40. We live in _____ of our own making and these
affect, relationships	self-made climates _____ our _____ with others.
conditions	41. Working _____ and an employee's percep- tions of those conditions affect individual
morale	_____ and determine the work climate.
collective	42. Organizational climate is the _____ view of the people within an organization as to the nature of the environment in which they work, and they can make that climate anything they want it to be.

CHAPTER 3—IMPROVED SUPERVISION THROUGH DELIBERATIVE LISTENING

	43. Bill Conboy has said that listening is a
skill	_____.
improved	44. Listening proficiency can be _____ with practice.
efficiency	45. Improved listening can mean greater _____ .

grievances

special

hear

analyze, recall

conclusions

45, talking

16

writing

check

receiving, sending

feedback

certified mail

five

six

like

positive

up

down

nonverbal

two

delivery

ideas, underlying

biases

fake

interrupt

46. Listening helps in settling _____ .

47. Listening makes people feel _____ .

48. Charles Kelly has defined deliberative listening as a unitary skill, the ability to _____ information, to _____ it, to _____ it at a later time, and to draw _____ from it.

49. Research shows that average working adults divide their communication time roughly along these lines: listening, _____ percent; _____, 30 percent; reading, _____ percent; and _____, 9 percent.

50. When something is extremely important, there is a need for a communication _____ .

51. If you defined communication with emphasis on the _____ end as well as the _____ end, you recognized the importance of listening.

52. The term _____ should be thought of as the "_____ _____" of communication.

53. There are _____ types of listening responses.

54. It has been suggested that each communicative act can involve at least _____ interpretations.

55. Normally one kind of behavior brings about a _____ behavior.

56. People tend to do something well when they hold _____ views or labels about their ability to do it.

57. There is a human tendency to live _____ or _____ to labels.

58. You should learn to watch for the speaker's _____ as well as verbal messages.

59. Everyone sends _____ messages.

60. You should not decide from a speaker's appearance or _____ that what he or she has to say is worthwhile.

61. You should listen for _____ and _____ feelings.

62. You should try to determine your own _____, if any, and allow for them.

63. Too many times people _____ attention.

64. You should not _____ immediately if you hear a statement that you feel is wrong.

word	65. You should not try to have the last _____.
500	66. Our minds function at _____ words per minute,
125	but we normally speak at _____ words per minute.
one-third, one-half	67. People forget _____ to _____ of what they
eight	hear within _____ hours.
	68. One technique that supervisors can use to improve their listening ability is to _____ that they
pretend	will be quizzed later in the day about what they have heard.

CHAPTER 4—IMPROVED SUPERVISION THROUGH ACTIVE LISTENING

easiest	69. Good listening habits are not the _____ of skills to develop, and that is why we may do it
poorly	so _____ .
sets	70. Too many times we develop mental _____ or
preconceived	_____ ideas as to what is being said.
	71. We hear the other person, but we are not
listening	_____ .
	72. Sometimes we fail to recognize that feelings
words	are not articulated by _____ .
intense	73. To be a good listener requires _____ concentration.
ears	74. We should listen with more than our _____ .
	75. Good active listening requires that we listen
all	for _____ possible meanings.
	76. To be effective the supervisor must listen
feedback	for _____ .
	77. One of the major barriers to interpersonal
judge	communication is our tendency to _____ what has been said.
55	78. Mehrabian found that _____ percent of the message is transmitted facially.
	79. When you actively listen, do not just word
swap	_____ .
	80. The second dimension of perception checking
parasupporting	is _____ .
much	81. Most of us talk too _____ .
	82. Most of us frame questions to get the answers
hear	we want to _____.

atmosphere s

facts

senses

83. Most of us set up communication in counter-productive _____ .

84. Most of us listen only for _____ .

85. Sometimes it is best to lose your mind and come to your _____ .

CHAPTER 5—THE DYNAMICS OF SUPERVISORY LEADERSHIP

leadership

1,800

group dynamics
social

two
task
individual

done

exclusive
four

high, high
high, low
high
low, low
low

high
high

loyalty, pride

Persuasive
arbitrary

86. In order to meet group goals, we must have _____ .

87. There have been more than _____ studies of leadership, but there is still little agreement on how to describe, identify, or evaluate it.

88. The concept of _____ _____ emerged from the _____ sciences.

89. Andrew Halpin notes that there are _____ main components of leadership: _____ behavior and _____ behavior.

90. The task oriented leader is mainly interested in getting the job _____ .

91. It should be remembered that the dimensions of task and individual behavior are not mutually _____ .

92. There are only _____ possible leadership behaviors.

93. The four leadership behavior patterns are: _____ task and _____ individual behavior, _____ task and _____ individual behavior, _____ individual and _____ task behavior, _____ task and _____ individual behavior.

94. Research studies indicate that employees derive a higher level of job satisfaction when their leaders exhibit _____ task and _____ individual behavior.

95. High-production groups show greater group _____ and greater group _____ than do low-production groups.

96. _____ climates tend to reduce tension and satisfy personal needs more than _____ climates.

trait	97. One of the earliest approaches in selecting leaders was called the _____ approach.
different, followers	98. R.M. Stogdill found that leaders could not be too much _____ from their _____ .
static	99. The trait approach examined only the _____ characteristics of leadership.
process	100. Leadership should be thought of as a _____ .
work	101. Successful managers manage _____
people	instead of _____ .
forget	102. Effective leaders often _____ about a problem for a while in order to solve it.
situation	103. Leadership effectiveness is dependent upon the _____.

CHAPTER 6—THE SUPERVISOR'S USE OF NONVERBAL COMMUNICATION

inflection	104. You communicate nonverbally through the _____ in your voice, your tone, your pitch;
gestures, facial	you use _____ and _____ expressions to communicate a whole range of meanings to the people you interact with.
proxemics	105. The study of distance is called _____ .
congruent	106. When the verbal and the nonverbal messages are _____ , we tend to have clear, meaningful communication.
dependent	107. Body language and spoken language are _____ upon each other.
55	108. Birdwhistell tells us that _____ percent of the social meaning in a conversation is transmitted nonverbally.
credibility	109. Nonverbal behaviors normally have a high degree of source _____ in the mind of
beholder	the _____ .
face	110. The _____ is the most reliable of all the nonverbal indicators.
second	111. Remember that paralanguage (voice inflection) is the _____ highest nonverbal indicator.

bodily

threatening

bubble

three

3, 20
20
5, 5
100

social

guess
probability

112. To a large extent, people's social identities and self-images are created by their _____ actions.

113. Touching is potentially the most _____ type of nonverbal behavior.

114. Personal space can be thought of as a plastic _____ that surrounds the individual.

115. According to Hall, there are _____ major interpersonal distances that govern our interpersonal relationships.

116. Intimate distance is from _____ to _____ inches, social distance from _____ inches to _____ feet, and public distance from _____ to _____ feet.

117. Nonverbal behavior must be interpreted in its proper _____ context.

118. Always remember that you abstract nonverbal meaning and that it is only an educated _____ with degrees of _____ .

CHAPTER 7—THE DYNAMICS OF THE SUPERVISOR'S WORK GROUP

collection

Delete
changes

pressure
agendas
group norm

norms

highly

norms, changed

pressure

119. A group is a _____ of individuals who affect the character of the group and who in turn are affected by the group.

120. _____ one member from a group and that group _____ in character.

121. Task-oriented groups usually operate under great _____ and have rigidly controlled _____ .

122. A _____ _____ may be defined as the shared acceptance of a rule.

123. The leader plays a key role in establishing the group _____.

124. Social pressure is highest in groups that are _____ cohesive.

125. Group _____ can be _____ but this is a difficult task.

126. Solomon Asch conducted an experiment to examine the effects of group _____ on individual judgment.

size	127. To a large extent, the effectiveness of a group is dependent upon its _____ .
five	128. Optimum size for small-group efficiency is _____ .
75	129. Robert Bostrom notes that in a five-man group there are a possible _____ interactions.
circular	130. A seating arrangement in a _____ pattern in which everyone can be seen may help to create a more open and friendly atmosphere.
four	131. There are _____ main communication networks.
wheel	132. The _____ allows the central person to communicate with any group member, and in turn the members must direct all their comments through the center.
chain	133. One of the major weaknesses of the _____ is that it lends itself to distortion.
chain	134. The _____ is normally used by organizations for the downward flow of information.
want	135. Subordinates tend to tell their supervisors what they think their supervisors _____ to hear.
wheel, chain	136. The _____ and the _____ are the best communication networks when the problem is
simple	_____ .
circle	137. The _____ lends itself to high participation and usually results in high group-member satisfaction.
star	138. Most authorities agree that in the majority of cases, the _____ pattern is the most suitable.
all-channel	139. The star pattern is sometimes called the _____ _____ network.
star	140. Member satisfaction appears to be highest in the _____ pattern.

CHAPTER 8—THE EFFECTIVENESS OF THE SUPERVISOR'S WORK GROUP

people	141. As a supervisor you are in the _____ business.
Meetings	142. _____ can be a useful tool; they are essential in order to impart information to or gain information from others.

ten

143. Executives typically spend an average of _____ hours a week in formal committee meetings.

7,000

144. The average executive spends almost _____ hours a year in meetings.

six

145. Jack Gibb developed _____ categories of behaviors that arouse defensiveness and ultimately affect the climate of the meeting or conference.

evaluation

146. To question one's values, standards, or beliefs is called _____ .

unannounced

147. A hidden agenda may be thought of as a person's _____ motives and intentions.

stoppers

148. The statements "that's ridiculous" and "we tried that before" should be seen as communication _____ .

discourage

149. These types of responses _____ group members from presenting new or different ideas.

pecking order

150. The solidified pattern of communication is commonly referred to as the communicative _____ _____ .

decision-making

151. The supervisor must involve the group in the _____ _____ process.

disagree
disagreeable

152. Effective groups have a tendency to_____ without being _____ .

dislike

153. Too often we associate disagreement with personal _____ .

permissiveness

154. Effective groups tend to have a high degree of _____ .

ineffective

155. Members of _____ groups act restrained during meetings.

skills, interests

156. Effective groups assign tasks on the basis of people's _____ and _____ .

status

157. To be effective as a group, there is a need for intergroup _____ .

successes

successes

158. To be effective, groups need _____ , and from _____ the group builds confidence and is able to meet new challenges.

CHAPTER 9—BARRIERS TO SUPERVISORY EFFECTIVE-NESS

language, abstrac-tions, sets

159. Our use of _____ , our _____ , and our mental _____ cause us not only to mislead others but, at times, to be misled by others.

two

160. It takes _____ to miscommunicate, and at times we deceive ourselves.

semantics
meaning
symbol
referent

161. A special area of study called _____ is concerned with the _____ of words, that is, the relationship between a _____ and the thing it represents, called a _____ .

signs, symbols

162. We use both _____ and _____ to communicate.

indicate, represent

163. An important distinction between the two is that signs _____ and symbols _____ .

humans
animals

164. The use of symbols is one of the basic characteristics that separates _____ from _____ .

shortcuts

165. Symbols may be thought of as communication _____ .

600,000

166. There are _____ words in the English language today.

influence
mean
meaning

167. Our past experiences determine which words have the most _____ in the communicative message and what they _____ to us.

168. When we believe that words have _____ , we are in serious trouble.

person

169. Words do not mean; the meaning is in the _____ .

vessels

170. If you think of words as _____ , then you are likely to talk about the meaning of a word as if the meaning were in that word.

verbal, situational

171. A supervisor must be able to differentiate between the _____ and _____ contexts of messages.

referents

172. Our communication problems are compounded when we both have the same meaning for the symbol, but different _____ .

Technical

173. _____ language was developed to facilitate quick and easy interpretation of messages between employees.

specificity

174. Symbols sometimes lack the needed degree of _____ for concise communication.

175. To communicate effectively, both parties must have the same communicative _____ .

code

abstracting
selectively

176. As communicators, we are constantly _____ information _____ .

177. We select bits and pieces of information based on our _____ , needs, and _____ .

feelings, attitudes

178. People allow us to see the person they want us to _____ .

see

deceived

179. We allow ourselves to be _____ .

180. How accurately you interpret messages is determined by your _____ .

abstractions

181. Always recognize that you are _____ and that these _____ may develop into mental _____ that limit your ability to see _____ .

abstracting
abstractions
sets, truth

182. There is a natural inclination to abstract results in a distorted perception of _____ by those who are accepting the information as _____ .

reality

gospel

183. A supervisor should never ask employees if they _____ , but rather _____ they _____ .

understand, what
understand
repeat

184. In this instance, the employees have to _____ what they have heard to the satisfaction of the supervisor.

185. Sometimes we think too much; we should use our _____ side in order to break mental sets.

sensing

sense

186. You have got to have good _____ in order to solve problems.

187. The goal of every communicative act is the _____ of a common meaning between the _____ and _____ of the message.

transfer
sender, receiver

CHAPTER 10—HOW TO INTERVIEW: THE FIRST STEP TO BETTER PLACEMENT

supervisor
planning

188. The final responsibility for hiring must lie with the employee's immediate _____ .

189. The interview requires advance _____ .

four	190. The interview has _____ major purposes.
information evaluate, information friend	191. The four purposes are: to get _____ , to _____ the applicant, to give _____ , and to make a _____ .
half	192. During the interview, the applicant should talk more than _____ the time.
4	193. Most personnel interviewers make their decisions after just _____ minutes of a 15-minute interview.
rapport	194. It is essential that you establish _____ with the candidate, who is often apprehensive about the interview.
Leading	195. _____ questions often move candidates to give the answers that they think the interviewer wants.
Probing	196. _____ questions are incisive and specific questions used to obtain more detail about a specific activity or area.
advance	197. It is a good idea to prepare your questions in _____ of the interview.
two	198. Supervisors often forget that there are _____ decisions to be made in every interview.
abruptly positive	199. The inexperienced supervisor will often end an interview _____ and many times on less than a _____ note.
stereotype	200. Do not _____ your interview.
overhire ability	201. Do not _____ , that is, do not select someone whose _____ far exceeds that required by the job.
formal	202. Do not be overly _____ .
advice	203. Do not give _____ to the applicant.
biases interview	204. Know your _____ and do not let them interfere with the _____ process.
screening	205. A _____ interview is useful when many applicants are applying for the same job.
letters reference	206. Do not pay too much attention to _____ of _____ carried by the applicant.

CHAPTER 11—EMPLOYEE MOTIVATION THROUGH IMPROVED SUPERVISION

motivate
behaviors
themselves
catalyst

three
caused
directed
motivated
inseparable
Maslow
motivational
Maslow
hierarchy
ladder

esteem

self-actualization

belongingness, es-
teem
humanistic

production
relationships

quality

closest

trigger

see
act
communication
empathic

207. No one can _____ another. All one can hope to do is to exhibit _____ that help others to motivate _____ .
208. A supervisor's behavior can act as a _____ to help employees motivate themselves.
209. There are _____ basic motivational premises.
210. Behavior is _____ .
211. Behavior is _____ .
212. Behavior is _____ .
213. Theory and practice are _____ .
214. The early work of _____ still serves as the main source of _____ theory today.
215. _____ contended that we are motivated by a _____ of human needs.
216. This hierarchy takes the shape of a _____ .
217. The fourth rung of this ladder represents our _____ needs.
218. The top rung of the ladder represents our need for _____ .
219. Research indicates that most employees are motivated by supervisors who stress the _____ and _____ needs of their employees.
220. The organizational climate in Japan is centered around concepts of _____ psychology which indicate that human relations are just as important as _____ .
221. The Japanese believe that the _____ between workers and management will be reflected in the _____ of goods and services.
222. Japanese managers and supervisors expect change and initiative to come from those _____ to the problem rather than from top administrators.
223. The words we use in our self-talk _____ pictures in our minds.
224. Deborah Briley believes that, as we _____ ourselves, so do we _____ .
225. Better supervisors tend to be _____ minded.
226. Better supervisors tend to be _____ listeners.

ask, persuade

227. Better supervisors tend to _____ or _____ rather than tell or demand.
228. High job satisfaction and quality work depend upon the maximum use of the individual work-

training, skill

er's _____ and _____ .
229. Employees can be motivated only through the

sharing, exertion

_____ of power, not through the _____ of power by a supervisor.

needs

230. People may be motivated by several _____ at the same time.
231. When employees feel dissatisfied, it is usually because they feel they are not being wisely

experience, training

utilized based on their _____ and _____ .
232. Most motivational theorists will tell you

money

that _____ is not a long-lasting motivator.
233. If there is one trait that separates average from exceptional human beings, it is that

positively

exceptional human beings talk _____ to themselves.
234. Exceptional persons hold themselves in high

esteem, dream

_____ and are not afraid to _____ .

enthusiasm

235. Nothing is ever accomplished without _____ .

fear

236. Sometimes _____ holds us back.
237. Your vision is the promise of what you shall

be

one day _____ .
238. Into your hands will be placed the exact result

thoughts

of your _____ .

seedlings

239. Dreams are the _____ of reality.

earn

240. You will receive that which you _____ ; no more, no less.
241. Whatever your present environment may be,

thoughts

you will fall, remain, or rise with your _____ , your vision, your ideal.

About the Authors

HARRY E. MUNN, JR.,is an associate professor of organizational communication at North Carolina State University in Raleigh. He received his bachelor of science degree from the University of Wisconsin and his master of arts degree in speech communication from Bradley University. His Ph.D., in speech communication and human relations, is from the University of Kansas.

Prior to teaching at North Carolina State University, he taught at Kent State University, the University of Florida, Miami-Dade Community College, and the University of Kansas.

He has written extensively in health care journals and is on the editorial board of *Hospital Topics*. He is the author of the *Nurse's Communication Handbook*. He is a consultant to a wide range of national and regional health care organizations. He has spoken to,. and participated in, seminars for nursing groups, hospitals, clinics, and health care associations from coast to coast.

NORMAN METZGER is vice president of Mount Sinai Medical Center in New York City, responsible for labor relations and personnel administration. He is director of the League of Voluntary Hospitals and Homes of New York City and was formerly president of that multiemployer association, which negotiates labor contracts for the voluntary hospitals in New York City. He is a professor of administrative medicine at the Mount Sinai School of Medicine; a professor in the graduate program in health care administration at Baruch College, the City University of New York; as well as a professor in the graduate program in health services administration at the New School for Social Research.

Mr. Metzger's experience in the labor arena spans 30 years in both the health services sector and in industry. He is the author or coauthor of six books and close to 100 articles in health care journals. He is a three-time recipient of the Literature Award of the American Society for Hospital Personnel Administration.

Index

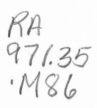